DATE DUE

MAY 3 0 1994	
OCT 1 3 1994	
Jan 16	
NOV 3 0 1998	
MAR 3 1 1999	
945032.	

BRODART   Cat. No. 23-221

Disease-Mongers

*How Doctors, Drug Companies, and
Insurers Are Making You Feel Sick*

Disease-Mongers

How Doctors, Drug Companies, and Insurers Are Making You Feel Sick

Lynn Payer

John Wiley & Sons, Inc.
New York • Chichester • Brisbane • Toronto • Singapore

Library of Congress Cataloging-in-Publication Data:

Payer, Lynn.
    Disease mongers : how doctors, drug companies, and insurers are
making you feel sick / Lynn Payer.
        p.   cm.
    Includes bibliographical references and index.
        ISBN 0-471-54385-3 (cloth)
        1. Medical ethics. 2. Physician and patient. 3. Medical care—
United States. 4. Insurance, Health—United States. I. Title.
    R724.P29   1992
    362.1'042—dc20   92-12513

Acknowledgments

I would like to thank Kerr White, M.D., Philip Caper, M.D., Nortin Hadler, M.D., Thomas Pickering, M.D., Eric Martin, M.D., Leonard Sigal M.D., and Gunnar B. Stickler, M.D. for critiquing an early draft of the manuscript and for helping me to shape this book in general. Any errors are, however, my own. I also appreciate the ideas about disease shared with Robert Hudson, M.D., over the years. In addition, I would like to thank everyone who agreed to give me time for an interview and who sent me materials.

Thanks to the staff of the Augustus C. Long Library at Columbia-Presbyterian Medical Center, where I spent many hours researching.

Thanks to my editor, Steve Ross, for seeing the potential in a book about "disease mongering," and for his suggestions throughout. Many thanks to my agent, Eleanor Wood, who has helped me shepherd a number of books through the publishing process, and to her children Kristina and Justin, who have put up with our numerous discussions over Chinese food.

A special appreciation to all those who have been supportive in a difficult time, especially my father and my sister. Thanks to Gwyn and Paul Kitos and their children, Peggy Weiss, Bill Williams, Brenda Jones, Gary and Irene Lincoff, Marcelle Arak, Virginia Payer, Karen McGinniss, Annie Desprez, Annie Bailleul, Josephine Markham, Annie Hoffman, and Evelyn Jacobs for providing frequent nurturance, both material and spiritual.

Contents

Foreword

The Publication of *Disease-Mongers* is particularly timely. In a medical marketplace that is becoming increasingly commercialized—and unaffordable—Lynn Payer's message is clear and simple: caveat emptor.

Concerns generated by rising health care costs, and the impaired access to medical care in both public and private sectors that has resulted from them, has prompted an increasingly intense examination of just what controls those costs. Purchasers of medical care have been experimenting with ways to handle the costs, and they are engaging in a much closer examination of the *value* of medical care services.

Early in this century, the evolution of medicine in much of the industrialized world was guided by the assertion (on the part of physicians) and the acceptance (on the part of policymakers, patients, and the general public) that modern medical care has a strong basis in scientific evidence. Decisions about whether to provide a particular test or treatment were thought to be determined by clear rules, based on scientific evidence, and applied more or less equally by different physicians. Given these assumptions, the discretion available to doctors and patients about treatment of a particular illness was thought to be minimal. Doctors were assumed to treat similar patients similarly. Each service was assumed to be "necessary." The quantity of medical care "required" by Americans would thus be determined by the amount of "real" illness in the American population, and would be self-governing.

But during the past fifteen years, evidence has been accumulating that much of medical decision-making is *not* firmly grounded in scientific evidence. Many medical practices are based more on anecdotal experience than scientific evidence, and treatment of the same illnesses are very different among physicians. Some physicians are much more aggressive than others in providing what is increasingly very expensive medical care. Yet, there is little evidence of any significant differences in the outcomes of the varying styles of practice, even though such differences lead to large discrepancies in costs.

We now have very convincing evidence that a large proportion of the rising costs of medical care are due to the *volume* of services being provided, rather than the *unit price* of each service. Furthermore, we are beginning to realize that the *amount* of medical care provided to individuals is, at best, only loosely related to the levels of actual illness. We must therefore begin raising questions about the *value* of the medical services we are receiving.

Is any slight potential decrease in morbidity and mortality due to aggressive diagnostic and treatment practices worth the cost? For most medical care, we cannot answer that simple question for two reasons. First, despite the impression of most medical consumers to the contrary, precise (and sometimes even approximate) information about the effectiveness of most medical care is simply not available. Without sound information about the effectiveness of medical services, cost/effectiveness measurements cannot be made.

Second, in addition to a dramatic rise in costs, the 1980s also saw an elevation in Americans' infatuation with the "marketplace." Marketplace economics have come to be viewed by some as the preferred way of controlling costs and improving quality. As a result, what used to be hospital services became product lines. What used to be services to the community became market share. What used to be nonprofit became for profit. The administrators of health care organizations came to be called presidents and CEOs. The MBA replaced the degree in public health as the credential of choice for growing numbers of health care executives. Competition—to get the largest number of patients through the door of whatever institution you worked for—became the aim of talented people filling the newly created posts of vice presidents for marketing. And patients became clients.

Because of the growing notion of medical care as a commercial rather than a public good, we have not yet decided whether such care is a right in America, and if so, how it is to be financed and distributed. Is everyone entitled to the same level of medical care, to a minimum level of care, or perhaps to no care at all if their illnesses are the result of socially condemned behavior or if they can't afford the costs? Should people be encouraged to purchase as much medical care as they want despite their real "needs," even if the medical services they consume could be better used by someone else?

In the absence of a consensus of those issues, it is impossible to place a *value* on the benefits of care, even if we could measure cost effectiveness precisely. A particular medical benefit may be worth a given price to a wealthy person, but not to a poor one, especially if the benefit is small relative to the price. If Americans decide that everyone should have access to the same medical care, we will value particular services differently than if we continue to treat medicine as a commodity that can be sold to the highest bidder.

Such is the current environment as skyrocketing medical costs, coupled with the progressive fragmentation of our system of financing medical services, have resulted in medical care being priced out of the reach of increasing numbers of middle-class working Americans.

In such a climate, publication of *Disease-Mongers* is particularly appropriate. In it, Ms. Payer examines some of the assumptions underlying the "medicalization" of many conditions and provides many persuasive examples. In other cultures, or perhaps in other times, many of these "diseases" would be treated as self-limited manifestations of the struggle of biological organisms, such as we humans against our heredity, the natural aging process, and the environment.

In contrast to that view, Americans seem to have an almost mystical belief in the effectiveness of modern "scientific" medicine in delaying or preventing illness and death. Until recently, cost has been no object in bringing these scientific forces to bear.

Due in part to this belief, the costs of medical care are now entirely out of control—driven by an increasing number of sophisticated tests and procedures that many experts believe diminish benefits. The use of increasingly expensive medical care for minimal or no benefit is exacting a heavy toll on those in our communities in the lower- to middle-income groups. The state of Oregon, for example, has found it necessary to propose explicit rationing of whole classes of medical care to some of its poorest citizens, in order to continue to provide what it considers basic services. The perceived need for such a program is driven entirely by the high costs of medical care.

Because of these trends, establishment of a higher level of accountability about how each of us—doctors and patients—use the medical care system is both desirable and inevitable. Questions such as those raised by Ms. Payer in this book are an important part of that process. She challenges us to go beyond questioning whether or not prescribed treatments are appropriate for our illness, and to ask, in addition, whether or not we are really sick at all!

In an open-ended system of financing medical care, such as that in the United States, it is becoming increasingly important for each of us—those ordering medical services as well as those consuming them—to become much more critical about how health care resources are deployed. In an environment as saturated with entrepreneurial zeal as the present-day health care system in America, a healthy dose of skepticism also seems to be in order. *Disease-Mongers* provides a good dose of that medicine.

PHILIP CAPER, M.D.
Professor of Public Policy, Dartmouth Medical School
Chairman, The Codman Research Group

Part One

How to Create Disease

Chapter 1

The Disease-Mongers

How the Medical–Industrial Complex Persuades You to Be Sick

Every well person is a sick person who doesn't know it.
—Jules Romains, *Knock.*

This man is seriously ill—and doesn't know it.
—Advertisement for a cholesterol-lowering drug.

When I read my paper, an ad (for "The Wellness Program") asks me if I have Silent Heart Disease, and when I turn on the TV, an ad (for Mazola oil) says, "I used to think my husband was healthy, but his doctor says his cholesterol is [dramatic sounds] *218!*" A news story in another paper quotes an American Cancer Society official who says that every American woman should consider herself at risk for breast cancer, while a press release (paid for by a drug company that promotes a drug for osteoporosis) that comes across my desk tells me that osteoporosis kills more women than breast cancer, although it doesn't say at what age. In the ladies' room at an airport a poster (undoubtedly funded—at least in part—by radiologists) tells me to have a mammogram. While fighting my way through a noisy and crowded Pennsylvania Station, I come across a small-time entrepreneur who wants to check my blood pressure; in return, I'm supposed to make a donation. On the subway coming home from a hard day at work, I'm confronted by a poster placed by a patient group that asks me to pick which of several normal-looking women has lupus; it then lists the symptoms, one of which is fatigue, with the implication that my fatigue might be due not to long hours of work and riding the subway but to lupus. Other posters ask if I have Aching Feet, which I probably do if I think about it, or Torn Earlobe, a possibility I had never even considered. And when I return home exhausted at 11 P.M., I have a message on my answering machine from a woman who has written a book about mitral valve prolapse, telling me that this condition, which I was once diagnosed as having, is not the benign condition we have been told, but really a serious disease. When I open the refrigerator door, a milk carton tells me that simply being over the age of 40 puts me at risk for diabetes.

Now I'm not a self-destructive person: I have never smoked, I limit my intake of alcohol, I exercise regularly, I fasten my seat belt, and I keep my weight within the bounds it should be for good health (depending, of course, on whom you listen to), if not for the latest fashions. I sometimes consult doctors. I enjoy comfort and freedom from pain at least as much as the next person.

But I have come to increasingly resent attempts to convince us that while we *think* we are well, we are *really* sick, riddled with all sorts of risk factors and anatomical abnormalities. We will all die sooner or later, and this gives the disease-mongers their insidious powers over us. But can the costly remedies promoted by the disease-mongers really postpone our dying? Can their remedies make us feel better? Can our money be better spent on something else? Are these messages really helping us? Or might they be hurting us?

In my 20 years as a medical journalist, I have become more and more convinced that much of the so-called information we get about our health grossly oversimplifies and distorts the reality. I know that both blood pressure and cholesterol readings are rough approximations of the risk of dying of heart disease. But I also know that the readings themselves vary greatly according to the conditions under which they are taken and that even the same reading means vastly different things depending upon your age, your sex, and various other risk factors. I also know there are studies showing that some people treated for mild hypertension are more likely to die than those who go completely untreated. I know that while four controlled studies have shown that screening mammography performed in women over the age of 50 does seem to cut the death rate from breast cancer, only one has shown any benefit in women under 50, something never acknowledged in the publicity urging women to get mammograms. I know that while osteoporosis may be a significant problem in older women, sometimes triggering a series of events that leads to death, it kills at a fairly advanced age, and everyone eventually has to die of something. And I know that even if my diagnosis of mitral valve prolapse had been correct, such diagnoses are pretty meaningless, since the consequences of the condition can vary from severe to none at all.

Perhaps most importantly, I realize that the most-heralded advances of modern medicine are simply mimicking what the healthy body does all by itself. While more people are now living to old age, there is no evidence that the maximum human life span has changed since biblical times, and some of the overall improvement may be due to natural selection, not medical intervention. As Thomas McKeown wrote in his book *The Role of Medicine: Dream, Mirage or Nemesis?:* "Like other living things, man has been exposed to rigorous natural selection, and the large majority of those born alive are healthy in the sense that they are adapted to the environment in which they live." Modern medicine may have a lot to offer the sick, but it should proceed with caution when dealing with the healthy.

But disease mongering—trying to convince essentially well people that they are sick, or slightly sick people that they are very ill—is big business. For people to use a diagnostic product or service, they must be convinced that they MAY BE sick. And to market drugs to the widest possible audience, pharmaceutical companies must convince people—or their physicians—that they ARE sick.

Disease mongering is the most insidious of the various forms that medical advertising, so-called medical education, and information and medical diagnosis can take. A doctor can advertise that he or she has just opened an office in the neighborhood, and that advertising informs us. A drug company can advertise that its pill is better than the pill of another drug company, and while this message may or may not be correct, it is at least not an effort to convince well people that they really are sick. But to tell us about a disease and then to imply that there is a high likelihood that we have it, either by citing the fact that huge numbers of Americans do (and who are we to escape?) or by citing symptoms such as fatigue that are universal and normal, is to gnaw away at our self-confidence. And that may make us really sick.

Take, for example, the case of a 37-year-old man who told his new doctor, "I was fine until a year ago when I found out that my cholesterol was high." This man really did have high cholesterol—300 mg/dL—and therefore was at a greater risk of having a heart attack than a man whose cholesterol was 200. But a heart attack was certainly not inevitable, particularly since he had no other risk factors; according to data from the Framingham study of cardiovascular risk, a man with his risk profile had a 6 to 7 percent chance of developing coronary heart disease in the following eight years. And there's no good evidence that by lowering his cholesterol—particularly with drugs—he would decrease his chances of dying an early death, since many studies have shown that while lowering cholesterol decreases death from heart disease, it *increases* deaths from other causes by about the same amount. The man tried dieting, but this failed to bring down his cholesterol, and he was put on lovastatin, a cholesterol-lowering drug. The patient stopped the drug because it made him feel terrible. According to Allan S. Brett, M.D., of Harvard Medical School, writing in the *American Journal of Medicine,* "He then stopped his daily exercise because of the fear that exercise would precipitate a heart attack," precisely the opposite of what someone with high cholesterol ought to do. "Finally, he had an episode of chest pain and tingling in the arms that led to a hospital admission to rule out myocardial infarction [heart attack]. A workup proved negative, and he was discharged with a diagnosis of hyperventilation. He now complains of insomnia." This man, who had previously been well, was now sick.

While the Food and Drug Administration (FDA) regulates claims made by drug companies about their drugs, disease mongering has been essentially unregulated, and FDA rules have actually favored its practice. A drug company, for example, cannot advertise the name of a drug to either the medical profession or the general public without giving a list of its known side effects, which for most drugs is quite extensive. But the company *can* place an ad implying that large numbers of people have the disease for which the drug is used and advising them to see their doctor, hoping that this will result in the doctor's prescribing the company's product. Because the drug industry also funds much of the postgraduate education that doctors get, the doctor probably will. While the new FDA head, Dr. David Kessler, has begun to take a harder look at some of these promotional practices, it's still unclear how much he will be allowed to regulate them.

Disease mongering has been around for a long time, and Americans have been particularly susceptible, partly because of our love affair with diagnosis and diagnostic tests. Our belief in the sanctity of diagnosis has led to a reimbursement system that depends on it (in contrast, as we shall see, to reimbursement systems in other countries). In a sort of chicken-and-egg scenario, making reimbursement dependent on diagnosis has reinforced the reverence paid to diagnosis while at the same time undermining its validity: 60 percent of the problems seen by primary care physicians don't fit into neat labels, but under our reimbursement system the doctor must write down *something*, right or wrong. Hospitals buy computer programs to help them assign the diagnosis that will pay the most. As journalist Jeff Schmidt was told by his doctor's receptionist when he asked if his insurance would cover a routine physical, "The doctor will provide you with sufficient diagnoses."

WHY AMERICANS ARE PARTICULARLY SUSCEPTIBLE

Perhaps one reason we Americans have become susceptible to disease mongering is that we lack the forceful images of disease-mongering characters found in the literature of other lands. England had George Bernard Shaw's Cutler Walpole, for example, who made himself ridiculous by diagnosing everyone as having a putrefying nuciform sac that should be removed, and today the Thames TV character Shelley talks of diseases manufactured to meet the need of the latest pills. France can remember some of Molière's more colorful characters, whose hypochondria was exploited by their doctors.

In the early part of this century, Jules Romains's Dr. Knock, whose motto was that every well person was simply a sick person who didn't know it, captured the French imagination, and this classic parable about what social scientists call "medicalization" is still taught in French high schools. In the play, Dr. Knock purchases a practice in a small French town where, while nearly everyone suffers from rheumatism, they would no more think of seeing a doctor about it than of going to the priest to cry. As a result, the doctor from whom Knock bought the practice wasn't terribly prosperous. Dr. Knock quickly establishes alliances with the sources of information—the schoolmaster, whom he instructs to inform the people about the dangers of germs, and the town crier, who announces that the doctor will be giving free consultations. At the consultations, at which Knock determines whether his patients are able to pay and how much ("That will cost you approximately two pigs and two steers"), he begins diagnosing frightening-sounding conditions that convince his patients that they must be under his care every day, often in bed, depriving themselves of everything but water. At the end of the play, the town is completely medicalized, with all the people under Knock's instructions, taking their temperatures all at the same time, several times, every night. Not only does Knock prosper, but so do the town hotel, which has become a hospital, and the town pharmacist. When you refer to Knockism today in France, everyone knows exactly what you are talking about.

By contrast, most literary and TV images of physicians in the United States range from benign to angelic, and when fault *is* found, it is usually for missing the diagnosis, not for finding disease where there is none. Dorothy, of the "Golden Girls" television series, for example, travels from doctor to doctor until she finally is given the satisfaction of a diagnosis of chronic fatigue syndrome, not seeming to realize that this diagnosis simply means that someone has been tired for a long time and nobody knows why. The doctor, played by William Hurt in the movie of that title, tells his fellow patient that her brain tumor would most certainly have been diagnosed by a magnetic resonance imaging (MRI) scan that the insurance companies were too chintzy to pay for, failing to clarify that even if diagnosed, many brain tumors are still incurable. One classic acknowledgment of disease mongering occurred on the television series "Doctor, Doctor," where Mike's plastic surgeon aunt suggests that General Manuel Noriega would have turned out nicer if only he'd had dermabrasion.

WHY DISEASE MONGERING IS INCREASING

But while there has always been a certain amount of disease mongering, social and economic conditions in America today make the practice particularly fierce.

• *There are too many doctors for too few patients.* The number of doctors has increased much more rapidly than the population over the past 20 years, thus giving each doctor fewer patients upon whom to make a living. While on paper the United States doesn't have more doctors per capita than the countries in Western Europe, American doctors are all competing for a limited portion of the American population: those who have insurance of some kind. With 35.7 million (and rising) Americans currently without health insurance, that portion is decreasing.

Specialists are fighting with other specialists over the right to treat certain types of disease, such as coronary artery disease, and in the process people with milder and milder disease—disease so mild that the treatment may pose more risks than the disease itself—are being diagnosed and treated. All these doctors must learn how to do the procedures on someone, and one cardiologist suggested that the ideal patient to practice on was one who probably didn't need the operation in the first place.

If the demand for medical care were well defined, competition might work to the advantage of the patient, making doctors cheaper and nicer. Certainly there are many doctors practicing who try to be honest with their patients; these doctors usually report spending a lot of time convincing their patients that they don't have the latest disease they heard about on TV or in the newspaper. But on the whole, more doctors, who have medical school loans to pay off and families to raise, will simply make more disease, particularly when most insurance companies will pay for a consultation only if there is a diagnosis given and will pay more for diagnostic tests than for time spent talking to patients.

• *Doctors are scared to death of being sued for malpractice.* They perceive that juries will be much harder on sins of omission (failing to diagnose a disease that is there) than sins of commission (diagnosing a disease that isn't there, making the disease seem more serious than it really is, or harming patients by doing something to them). Doctors and laboratories are fearful that if they give a patient a clean bill of health and the patient later develops a disease, they may be liable for malpractice. This may be why my preoperative chest X-ray report was something like, "We can't see very much, but we have no reason to think that there's serious disease present." Gone are the days when a visit to the doctor could end with patients' learning they had nothing wrong with them.

• *There are many more popular health magazines and newspaper supplements than there used to be.* Often these are seen more as ways to draw advertising revenue than as serious journalism. Popular health tracts have been around since before the invention of the printing press, when they were copied by hand by monks. But the past decade has shown a mushrooming of news about health and illness, with many papers adding special sections and many new magazines starting. Some of them are pretty good. But others are simply seen as a way to increase advertising revenue, and they do this by running articles mongering diseases that the advertisers' products can be seen to prevent or treat.

• *Recent changes in the way hospitals are paid have given them incentives to "up" the severity of the diagnosis.* Hospitals used to be paid for whatever procedures they performed on patients, a system that gave them incentives to do as much as possible to each patient, regardless of diagnosis. They were also paid for the number of days the patients stayed, which gave them incentives to keep the patients in as long as possible. In an attempt to contain the rapid rise in health care costs, health economists devised a payment system based on the diagnosis, known as diagnosis-related groups, usually called DRGs.

The establishment of DRG was undoubtedly a good-faith effort to control costs, and as health economist Victor Rodwin, Ph.D., of New York University, points out, DRGs were the first attempt even to establish a dialogue as to how much care was appropriate for a given diagnosis. But the DRG system is based on the belief that diseases are "things"—the folly of which will be shown in chapter 2—and that diagnoses were much more cut and dried than they really are. A few physicians early on identified what was to be a major problem with the DRGs: there is a large amount of uncertainty in medical diagnosis and therefore considerable leeway as to whether you diagnose something as disease A or disease B. If disease B pays the hospital more, the hospital will attempt to get doctors to make diagnosis B rather than diagnosis A. The DRG system also gives the hospitals incentives to recruit as many new patients as possible into the hospital, preferably ones that aren't too sick, since they will require less care.

The practice of assigning a slightly more serious diagnosis was baptized "DRG creep" by D. W. Simborg, one of the doctors who early on recognized its abuse potential. But by the late 1980s, some of the DRGs seemed to be leaping rather than creeping: Susan Horn, Ph.D., of Johns Hopkins University, found when looking through hospital records that a number of patients with the diagnosis of myocardial infarction (heart attack) or shock showed absolutely no signs of having these diseases.

While health economists debate the implications of DRG creep (or leap) on hospital financing, most seem not to have considered that it can also have major implications for any individual who has to apply for insurance, as these inflated diagnoses can become a part of the medical records used by insurance companies to deny insurance or to contest payment on the basis that the person lied about a preexisting condition. One wonders, for example, what will happen to the man coded as having a heart attack even though he didn't if he must change his medical insurance plan or employment for some reason.

• *The pharmaceutical industry's role in postgraduate medical education has increased dramatically.* From 1975 to 1988, the drug industry's funding of symposia increased fourteenfold. While some of the more flagrant practices of drug promotion, such as giving doctors frequent-flier points every time they prescribe a particular drug, are coming under criticism, the so-called educational activities are usually lauded. Indeed, many medical seminars sponsored by drug companies are of a high quality. But drug companies nearly always have some say about the topic and about who is invited to speak, and most have a "stable" of speakers, none of whom is likely to say that a disease is not very important or that it should be defined very narrowly, since that would limit the amount of a drug that will be prescribed.

•   *Restraints on advertising have changed.* Restraints on physicians have broken down, and those on prescription drugs directly to consumers are in the process of dissolving. Some doctors are now advocating that patients be able to order their own diagnostic tests, and we can perhaps expect to see ads advising patients to come in for a Lyme disease test, for example. In theory, physician advertising was supposed to lead to price competition that would drive costs down. In practice, it has opened the doors to advertisements that convince more and more people that they are sick—that their leg pain, for example, may in fact be a sign of a serious illness—and costs continue to rise.

THE NEGATIVE EFFECTS

Disease-mongers consider that they benefit public health by identifying and treating more and more people who are ill. This is sometimes true. There are instances where early detection can lead to a treatment that cures an otherwise serious disease with relatively few side effects. But disease-mongers don't consider (or choose to ignore) the negative effects of convincing well people that they are sick. The negative side effects of disease mongering are numerous and daunting:

•   *Disease mongering exposes people to the physical risks of unnecessary testing, which occasionally proves fatal.* Angiography, for example, the examination of the coronary arteries by means of a catheter, leads to about one or two deaths for every 1,000 persons tested. About two of every 10,000 persons who undergo colonoscopy to screen for colon polyps—which may turn into cancer but again may not—will have their colon perforated, a situation that requires surgery with a 5 to 10 percent mortality rate. A routine investigation for patients with disorders of the biliary tract and pancreas causes pancreatitis—which can be fatal—in 2 to 5 percent; and at least one physician believes that AIDS was spread in Africa by malaria tests that were performed in an unsanitary manner. A small percentage of patients will have dangerous allergic reactions to the contrast media used in radiologic examinations, occasionally resulting in death. Every X-ray results in an increase in the total dose that a person receives in his or her lifetime, and the larger the total dose, the greater the risk that the radiation will cause a cancer.

• *Disease mongering exposes people to the risks of unnecessary treatment, and here, too, some may die.* Even tests as seemingly innocuous as a measurement of cholesterol or blood pressure may cause mischief if they are not used by a wise doctor. Both tests are notoriously inaccurate, and many people are told they have high cholesterol or blood pressure when they really don't. If treatment with drugs is started without repeat readings and without an assessment of whether the risks of the drugs will be greater than the risks of the high cholesterol or blood pressure, people may die of the treatment. Diabetics who are given diuretic drugs for their high blood pressure, for example, have a higher death rate than diabetics whose high blood pressure is untreated; and nearly all studies of cholesterol lowering, either with diet or drugs, show that while deaths from heart attack decrease, deaths from other causes rise. People given antibiotics for Lyme disease they don't really have will be at risk of allergic reactions, yeast infections, and gallstones; the promiscuous use of antibiotics will also increase the chances that the next time that person gets an infection, the antibiotics won't work. Women whose Pap tests are somewhat abnormal may be talked into a hysterectomy that is not necessary to save—and may decrease the quality of—their lives.

• *Disease mongering causes individuals, as well as society, to pay their health dollars for diagnoses and treatments of marginal value or no value at all.* At the same time we neglect other treatments that are cheaper and of unquestioned value. We in the United States pay 12 percent of our gross national product for health care, yet our life expectancy compares unfavorably with that of many countries in Asia and Western Europe, and many countries manage to spend less, yet achieve better results that are extended to the entire population. Disease mongering is a major contributor to this crisis. A firm that manufactures monitors supposed to detect premature labor (and which cost $5,000) can, by careful marketing, convince women, their doctors, and their insurance that the women must use the monitor, even though there's no evidence that detecting premature labor prevents premature births. Huge amounts of money are therefore spent for procedures of questionable benefit, while proven methods of preventing prematurity, such as reasonable prenatal care, particularly for poor women, often go begging.

• *Disease mongering often presents magical solutions to a problem, whereas in fact the problem may have only a partial solution.* The way mammography is being promoted as a solution to the problem of breast cancer, for example, often leaves the impression that if only women would get annual mammograms, they'd never get breast cancer, or at least not die of it. Such promotions don't emphasize that mammography lowers the death rate from breast cancer only by about one-third, and then only in some age groups. The focus on mammograms may cause women to neglect routine physical examinations, which may be more important in women under the age of 50, and seems to give some doctors the dangerous idea that they can give drugs that may increase the risk of breast cancer with impunity as long as they order mammograms.

• *Disease mongering exposes people to social discrimination.* People are routinely denied jobs and health and life insurance based on diagnoses, no matter how silly. One English doctor who offered free checkups found that the only patients who did not take the offer were insurance brokers who did not wish the doctor to have information that would be used against them by insurance companies. In England the situation is better than it is in the United States, since patients there do not have to worry about being denied health insurance.

Mary Ann Bailey and Dr. Philip Rosenthal, then of the Children's Hospital of Los Angeles, wrote to various U.S. insurance companies in an attempt to determine exactly what their policies were regarding the insurability of many gastrointestinal diagnoses given to children. Most companies refused to respond, and among those who did there was no agreement as to which conditions would cause insurance to be denied altogether, which would result in higher rates, and which would be insured at normal rates. While this may be comforting to someone denied insurance by one company, it points out the irrationality of the practice. Cleverly, Bailey and Dr. Rosenthal included in their list of diagnoses one that doesn't exist: chronic hepatitis A. Six of the eight companies said that a person with this diagnosis would be uninsurable!

In addition, privacy laws in the United States are particularly lax, meaning that such information, accurate or not, is difficult to hide; European countries often won't allow data to flow to the United States because of our failure to protect privacy. Dorothy Thompson, an English doctor practicing in the United States, wrote about a woman from an insurance company who routinely called her about patient diagnoses. "Apparently I am the only doctor she has ever met who refuses to give this information. If this is true, I despair of patient confidentiality in the United States."

According to Michael W. Miller, writing in the *Wall Street Journal*, physicians are often enticed to sell their medical records to drug companies and other medical groups. Supposedly, patient names are deleted, but with social security numbers, age and sex often a part of the record such patients could be identified, and if they are they don't have a great deal of legal recourse. According to Miller, "privacy law covers videotape rentals and cable-TV selections, but not most medical records." While some states have laws protecting confidentiality in the case of an AIDS diagnosis, an Ohio jury recently found that a hospital employee didn't violate any law when she allegedly discovered a friend's AIDS diagnosis in the hospital computer and told other hospital workers about it.

The situation may even be getting worse: recently when a doctor was unable to sell his practice to another doctor, a lay person bought the records and sold them back to the patients, and in 1991 a clinic treating AIDS patients provided patient lists to a politician running for office. David A. Testone, who used to sell health insurance for Mutual of Omaha and now works as a consultant for people with insurance problems, says that he was part of Mutual of Omaha's aptly named S.S.—special services— department that sought to find out if patients had been hiding any medical records. A patient who had been seeing a doctor for epilepsy but trying to keep it secret from the insurance company by not submitting any doctor bills might be tripped up, for example, by a check of the pharmacy to see which doctors had been writing prescriptions for that patient.

• *A diagnosis often adversely affects the quality of life, causing people to worry, which can lead to increased absenteeism, impaired sex life, and in some cases even suicide.* Abnormal Pap tests, for example, can be the source of considerable anxiety, causing changes in attitudes to sex and to sex partners, with decreased frequency of intercourse and decreased arousal and orgasm. These negative effects may persist even if the diagnosis was wrong and the patient is told it was wrong. Patients diagnosed as having high blood pressure and later "dediagnosed" reported more depression and a lower state of general health than a matched group not mistakenly diagnosed as hypertensive. Not only will worry impair the quality of life and lead to spending money on things that may not be of any real importance to health, but there's some evidence that worry about one's health may itself be a cause of sickness. "Angst and well-being simply cannot stand together," wrote John F. Burnum, M.D., in Annals of Internal Medicine.

Women who have second heart attacks tend to have been more anxious and fearful after the first than women who have just one, and a number of studies hint that breast cancer patients with a positive attitude live longer. Ellen L. Idler and Stanislav Kasl found that people's answer to the simple question "Is your health excellent, good, fair, or poor?" was a better predictor of who would live or die over the next decade than even a rigorous physical examination. While it could be that people are more sensitive to certain signs of mortality than are their doctors, it could also mean that telling people they are sick becomes a self-fulfilling prophecy, causing them to become sicker.

The placebo effect, by which people get better even when given a sugar pill because they believe they will get better, is a powerful component of both orthodox and alternative medicine, and the opposite of the placebo effect is the negative placebo or nocebo effect. Telling people they are sick undoubtedly has a strong negative placebo effect; and while disease-mongers may well argue that the remedies they are promoting counteract this negative placebo effect, it's a costly way to do things. In some cases, of course, a diagnosis, particularly of being positive on the "AIDS test," results in suicide, a particularly frightening possibility when one considers that these individuals didn't really have AIDS but simply tested positive for the HIV virus—a test that isn't 100 percent accurate.

There must be a balance between worrying too little about our health and worrying too much, and as a nation we seem to have crossed the line where we are probably worrying too much. "The individual's belief in his health is precious," wrote Thomas McKeown. "With a little injudicious prompting a cheerful extrovert can be transformed into a melancholy hypochondriac, and a whole community can become preoccupied with disease when undue emphasis is placed on its precursors. This trend is already evident in the United States and Canada."

As Arthur Barsky put it in *Worried Sick*: "We could become a nation of healthy invalids, crippled not by disease but by the idea of disease."

There is, in fact, a marked contrast between the messages we get about what we should do to be healthy and what some of the top physicians do, both for themselves and for their patients. Mark E. Josephson, M.D., a professor of cardiology at the University of Pennsylvania Medical School, told a symposium on arrhythmias at New York's Mount Sinai Hospital in the spring of 1989 that on his service the reliance was not on fancy tests. "To decide whether someone is going to die suddenly I listen to their heart and lungs and decide if they're sick. If they're sick, they're more likely to die than if they're healthy. I'll make a phone call every month and if they answer the phone then they're okay."

Another cardiologist, Thomas Pickering, M.D., a professor of medicine at New York Hospital-Cornell Medical Center, admits that he "has had the odd twinge of chest pain myself, but haven't done anything about it, because once getting into the system you don't know where it will lead."

Most of us, of course, don't have Dr. Pickering's level of knowledge in interpreting our symptoms, and we should see a doctor for significant ones such as chest pain. But as I hope to show in the following chapters, treatments, tests, and even diagnoses all have their risks. Rather than choosing the doctor who always gives a diagnosis, who performs lots of tests, and who treats aggressively, you may want to find one who knows that too much medicine can be as bad as not enough and who judiciously considers not only the benefits of each procedure but also its risks.

Chapter 2

A Disease Is Not a "Thing"

One of the most widespread diseases is diagnosis.
  —Karl Kraus, *Half-Truths and One and a Half Truths.*

Medical men all over the world having merely entered into a tacit agreement to call all sorts of maladies people are liable to, in cold weather, by one name; so that one sort of treatment may serve for all, and their practice thereby be greatly simplified.
  —Jane Welsh Carlyle, letter to John Welsh, March 4, 1837.

Colds, you know, are not the thing at all, up here; they are not *reçus*. The authorities don't admit their existence; the official attitude is that the dryness of the air entirely prevents them. If you were a patient, you would certainly fall foul of Behrens, if you went to him and said you had a cold. But it is a little different with a guest—you have a right to have a cold if you want to.
  —Thomas Mann, *The Magic Mountain,* 1924.

Politicians discovered long ago that a good way to pass the buck is to get a problem labelled as a disease.
  —Dr. Michael O'Donnell, *The Medical Post,* June 25, 1985.

Journalist Jeff Schmidt requested a stress test when he was in his forties because of a family history of heart problems. "I got my doctor to refer me for one at a nearby hospital, but when I got to the stress test department there, I found myself caught in a catch-22: I couldn't proceed with the 'diagnostic procedure' without first supplying a diagnosis. My referral slip—a small prescription sheet—did not mention any diagnosis, and so the aide in charge of the all-important paperwork asked me for one. When I said I didn't have one, he invited me to make one up so that they could go ahead with the test. To make this exercise in creativity easy for me, it would be multiple choice rather than fill in the blank. The form he was filling out offered more than a dozen choices, but none of them were appropriate for someone in my situation. When I had a hard time choosing, he suggested one: 'C.A.D. (ASHD).' This was a popular one, he informed me, but he didn't know what it stood for, and I didn't have a clue. I ended up choosing one that I could at least understand," he said, selecting arrhythmia (irregular heartbeat) as his choice.

This incident tells a lot about diagnosis in America today. By requiring a diagnosis in order to get test or treatment paid for, we are manufacturing more and more labels with less and less meaning. Such labels are then taken up by epidemiologists, who in turn try to make sense of "new" disease patterns. The labels are also sent to insurance companies, which keep them in a central data bank in Massachusetts. (See Chapter 18 for the address). Indeed, the same diagnosis that may help patients get reimbursed for screening tests may cause them to be denied health insurance if they must reapply, a situation happening with increasing frequency in today's sluggish economy and chaotic health insurance market. Susan Love, M.D., a breast surgeon and clinical professor at Harvard Medical School, points out that in order to help their patients get reimbursed for their screening mammograms, doctors may put down "fibrocystic disease" (a meaningless term as we shall see in Chapter 14). As a result, these women may later be denied insurance for anything having to do with their breasts—or denied coverage altogether on the basis of this diagnosis.

Many Americans assume that symptoms must be clear-cut signs of disease, and all they need is the right doctor to find the diagnosis. Magazine editors reinforce this notion by habitually (and often inaccurately) pointing out that "this symptom" inevitably means "that disease," an equation that makes for punchier copy and probably even a chart. Americans also seem to believe that finding the diagnosis will inevitably lead to a cure, as reflected in the popular saying "The first step to cure is diagnosis." Medical schools put a lot of emphasis on coming up with obscure diagnoses. Kerr White, M.D., recalls that when he was a young faculty member at the University of North Carolina in Chapel

Hill, everyone put money in a kitty, and the resident who came up with the most arcane diagnosis of the week would win the kitty. Doctors are paid more for performing diagnostic tests than for examining or talking to their patients. Juries hearing malpractice cases seem to consider missing a diagnosis one of the worst sins a doctor can commit (much worse than killing a patient by ordering too many diagnostic tests or by treating him or her too much). This unquestioned acceptance of, and reliance upon, diagnosis, however, obscures several points:

- Many "diagnoses" are simply descriptions of symptoms, often phrased in Latin or Greek to sound more important.
- A disease is not a "thing."
- There's no agreement in medicine on the definition of "disease."
- A diagnosis doesn't always help treatment.

Let's examine these points more closely, one at a time.

- *Many diagnoses are simply descriptions of symptoms.* If you tell the doctor that your muscles are sore, he or she may tell you that you have *myalgia*, which is Greek for muscle pain. *Cephalgia* is Greek for headache. If the conjunctiva, or mucous membrane that lines the eye, gets inflamed, you're likely to get a diagnosis of *conjunctivitis*, which is Latin for inflammation of the conjunctiva. This is probably why doctors used to have to learn Latin and Greek: Diagnoses sound much more important in a foreign language.

Patients, of course, often demand a diagnosis, and some studies have shown that a diagnosis itself has a powerful placebo effect, with patients frequently being satisfied that their illness has a name and not wanting any further treatment. In fact, wrote Samuel Vaisrub, M.D., in the *Journal of the American Medical Association*, "to them, diagnosis may be the most important part of therapy." So doctors cannot really be faulted for their habit of describing symptoms in Latin or Greek. It's just that doctors and patients both need to understand that this doesn't mean they have been "possessed" by an important-sounding desease, but simply that they have a symptom.

- *A disease is not a real "thing."* Most people think of diseases as "things" that somehow possess the body much as a devil might, and a diagnosis is seen as the first step toward exorcism.

According to E. J. M. Campbell, J. G. Scadding, and R. S. Roberts, writing in the *British Medical Journal*, "Most people without medical training seem to think of a disease as an agent causing illness." Doctors have a somewhat more complex view of diseases, they wrote, but doctors have a reason for sharing the patient's view, at least in part. "Naming a disease as the cause of a patient's illness may have a useful function in the doctor-patient relationship, especially the general practitioners: the disease becomes a third party, the real enemy."

The idea of diseases as "things" can be found in ancient Greek medicine, but it gained particular prominence in the work of Thomas Sydenham in the seventeenth century. Before Sydenham, doctors tended not to classify symptoms into diseases. Instead they recognized "humoral imbalances." Sydenham lived in the time when biologists were busy classifying plants and animals, and he attempted to classify diseases in the same way. With plants and animals there is an ultimate test of the concept of species: whether individuals can interbreed with one another. There is no such test for "diseases" (although there can be for the microbes that cause them, since microbes are tiny living things themselves).

Most philosophers of diagnosis now realize that diseases are not things, but are instead organizational concepts: the (sometimes arbitrary) ways in which doctors organize the signs and symptoms of illness as they occur in different people into something they can deal with, study, and make predictions about. In other words, your suffering (illness) is real, but "disease" is a construct, a classification in the head—in the doctor's head.

Doctors therefore do not "discover" diseases; they define them. If the criteria for certain diseases look as if they were designed by a committee, they usually are. Take, for example, the criteria for a diagnosis of systemic lupus erythematosus, an autoimmune disease that most commonly affects women: you have to have at least four symptoms from the list or it's not lupus. Other diseases are defined rather like ordering from a Chinese menu: take two symptoms from A and two from B. The need to place combinations of signs and symptoms into neat little packages has led to the concept of "overlap syndrome": diseases that don't fit into the definition but have many symptoms in common with other diseases. As I have shown in another book, *Medicine and Culture,* the definition of diseases often varies quite widely from one country to another: in the United States one seizure is considered sufficient for a diagnosis of epilepsy, while in England you have to have at least two. Some U.S. residents could "cure" their epilepsy simply by moving to England.

Other diseases are defined according to their duration. An editorial in the British journal the *Lancet,* for example, pointed out that how long you have to have symptoms in order to be given a diagnosis will depend on what disease you have. One panic attack, for example, can be sufficient to yield a diagnosis of panic attack, while to get a diagnosis of dysthymic disorder, you have to have depressive symptoms for most of the time during the previous two years. "The reasoning behind the time limits imposed on different diagnoses," wrote the editorialist, "is far from clear. The diagnosis of major depressive episode requires depressive symptoms to have been present for two weeks, but for its anxiety equivalent, generalised anxiety disorder, symptoms have to have been present for most of the previous six months to qualify for the diagnosis." This situation can lead to a doctor's saying, essentially, "Come back tomorrow, Mr. Smith. Today you fail to qualify for diagnosis, treatment, or insurance cover. Tomorrow, however, if your symptoms persist, I will be able to help you."

The concept of disease can be quite useful, as it frequently enables doctors to predict what will and will not work therapeutically. In some cases, diseases behave so predictably it's almost as if they *were* "things." But while disease concepts work well as long as they're understood to be hypothetical, people who view diseases as "things" get into problems.

Even with infectious diseases, which most nearly fit the concept of diseases that possess us, a lot of the form the disease takes depends upon the person in whom the disease occurs. Sydenham tried to get around this problem three centuries ago by separating the symptoms of "disease" from the symptoms unique to particular individuals with the disease, in an attempt to find what was universal in the disease as opposed to idiosyncratic signs of illness. But doctors today tend to play down or ignore these idiosyncratic elements in their emphasis on diagnosing and treating "diseases." This emphasis "has been damaging to medical thinking," according to Stanley Joel Reiser, M.D., an historian of medical philosophy writing in *Annals of Internal Medicine.* "Such a focus leads to a relative obscuring or ignoring of those elements of illness that are novel expressions of the patient's self, and to a homogenizing process that can cause physicians to downplay the patients' individuality and emphasize instead the patients' connections with populations."

One of the main problems, in fact, with the concept of diseases and with specific diagnoses is that they oversimplify. A disease always occurs in a particular person and will be different depending upon many things about that person. Since most diseases vary widely in their severity, doctors often break up diseases bearing the same name into stages or subtypes. Cancers, for example, are divided according to how extensively they have spread as well as the particular type of cell that is spreading. Even then, the cancer will often act differently depending upon other characteristics of the patient. The people who thought up the system of diagnosis-related groups (DRGs) as a way of paying for care are learning this the hard way. First there were DRGs, then there were severity-adjusted DRGs, and now people are attempting to refine payment further based on individual characteristics of the patients themselves, not of their diagnosis, in an attempt to figure out how much care a given patient needs.

But while physicians predicted this would happen, they, too, fall prey to the oversimplification produced by disease labels. One would assume that do-not-resuscitate orders would be written for patients who wanted them and would be directly related to the patients' prognosis—whether or not there was a chance that after resuscitation they would be able to have a reasonable quality of life. But investigators have found that doctors were much more inclined to write do-not-resuscitate orders for patients with certain diagnostic labels. While AIDS, lung cancer, cirrhosis, or severe congestive heart failure all have similar prognoses, investigators at the three teaching hospitals of the University of California at San Francisco found that do-not-resuscitate orders were written for 52 percent of patients with AIDS and 47 percent of patients with cancer, but for only 16 percent of patients with cirrhosis and 5 percent of patients with congestive heart failure.

• *There is no general agreement on the definition of "a disease."* According to J. G. Scadding, professor of medicine at the University of London and a leading philosopher of diagnosis, "the word 'disease' is in general use without formal definition, most of those using it allowing themselves the comfortable delusion that everyone knows what it means."

In spite of there being no definition of what a disease is, people spend valuable time debating whether a given condition is or is not a "disease." Since each disease is itself a definition, one can define what elements a given illness has to have to be considered a disease. But such debate has about as much practical value as debating how many angels can dance on the head of a pin—except when the reimbursement system demands that for something to be paid for, it must be a disease.

In general, says Robert Hudson, M.D., a medical historian at the University of Kansas Medical Center and author of *Disease and Its Control*, (Westport, CT: Greenwood) the definition of a disease has varied historically and across cultures. "Disease has always been what society chooses it to mean—neither more nor less." Common to most definitions, he says, are two elements: it usually implies some kind of impairment, and it's what doctors treat. "In desperation," he wrote, "someone defined disease as something people go to doctors for."

• *A diagnosis doesn't always help devise a treatment.* An editorial in the *Lancet* points out: "The importance of an accurate diagnosis in medicine may, in itself, be questionable. Although it has been a basic principle for over a century that one should establish the primary cause of a disease and treat it, intensive care units have shown that treatment of the effects of a disease rather than the disease itself can lead to recovery from serious illness by allowing the body to recover once chemical disturbances have been corrected. The need to put a name to the condition that one is treating seems to have more to do with the intellectual satisfaction of the doctor than the need of the patient." While intensive care units show that you don't always need a diagnosis for serious diseases, the fact that many people find their minor ailments are better cured by alternative medicines—which, if they depend on a diagnosis, use an entirely different process from that used by orthodox doctors—argues for nonspecific healing, which is often denigrated as the placebo effect.

In fact, the search for a diagnosis is often counterproductive to the real problem of the patient. Joseph D. Wassersug, M.D., a retired internist in Boca Raton, Florida, cites the case of an elderly man admitted to the hospital for a transient ischemic attack, who continually complained that he needed aspirin for his chronic headache. "The young doctor obtained skull X rays, an EEG, a CT scan, Doppler studies, arteriograms, and whatever else she could think of. Only after a battery of negative findings did she belatedly realize that the patient had been asking for aspirin and she'd ignored him. He got the aspirin, and the headache disappeared."

It is partly the primacy of diagnosis in American medicine that causes doctors to order so many tests. As Jerome Kassirer, M.D., who recently took over the editorship of the *New England Journal of Medicine*, points out, it is the American tendency to equate thoroughness with quality that results in so many tests being ordered. "Diagnostic certainty usually is unattainable; it is frequently not required for optimal care; and because all tests are imperfect and some impose risk, the attempt to reach certainty with more and more tests sometimes produces substantial harm."

THE ABUSE POTENTIAL OF DIAGNOSES

If you recall Dr. Hudson's statement that disease usually implies an impairment, and that it's something people go to doctors for, you can see the abuse potential. All sorts of things can be *perceived* as causing impairment: being too short, being too tall, having a difficult complexion, having slightly maloccluded teeth, or partially occluded blood vessels. As the American Society of Plastic and Reconstructive Surgeons argued in 1982, "There is a substantial and enlarging body of medical opinion to the effect that these deformities (small breasts) are really a disease which in most patients results in feelings of inadequacy." But the same condition that one person sees as an impairment may be seen by another as being an advantage. A short woman, for example, may be disadvantaged when reaching for something on a high shelf but advantaged in a culture that considers that women should be shorter than the men they date.

Clifton K. Meador, M.D., an endocrinologist at the University of Alabama College of Medicine who originated the term "nondisease", cites the case of a 20-year-old daughter of Italian parents who was referred for evaluation of "excessive facial hair" that caused the doctors to suspect an adrenal tumor. The mother and two sisters of the patient were also found to have "excessive facial hair" but commented that in their culture it was considered a mark of womanhood. A dermatologist once wanted to prescribe a cortisone cream for what he called my "acne rosacea" or tendency to flush under stress, presumably because he felt it must be distressing me; my friends, on the other hand, compliment me on my "good color." When a World Health Organization group tried to agree on a definition of orthodontic "disease" in order to find out how prevalent it was in the world, they were unable to, finally defining orthodontic disease as anything a trained orthodontist says it is. In the discussion at the close of the meeting, the participants admitted that "One set of figures quoted showed that the range of malocclusion in various populations extended from 50 percent in the Bantus to over 90 percent in Navaho Indians. This raises the question of whether malocclusion is in fact an abnormality at all. Many deviations from normal dental arrangements are aesthetically more satisfactory than regular dentitions resulting from orthodontic, prosthetic, or cosmetic restorative dentistry."

With a surplus of doctors looking for work, a pharmaceutical industry anxious to market new drugs, and a stable of medical writers looking for story ideas, there will be a tendency to perceive biologic disadvantage even where the patient doesn't feel particularly disadvantaged.

A GERM IS NOT A DISEASE

While there's no hard-and-fast definition of disease, in practice what doctors have traditionally considered disease falls into four major types.

The first type is the infectious diseases, and these fit most neatly into the category of "things." Indeed, something—a virus, rickettsia, bacteria, protozoa, or fungus—infects us, leading to symptoms that the doctor diagnoses as "disease." But it's important to realize that the germ is not the disease. Many germs infect us without usually leading to any disease at all: we all have strains of the bacterium *E. coli* in our gut and it causes diseases only if it gets into other areas of the body (and then only sometimes). Some germs are problems only if they infect us at certain vulnerable periods: infections with *Toxoplasma gondii* and rubella, for example, are usually minor for a healthy adult but can injure a fetus in the womb. Sometimes the same germ is associated with more than one disease: the same virus that causes chickenpox when it first infects us can lie dormant in a nerve, causing herpes zoster when it is reactivated years later; and Epstein-Barr virus is associated with infectious mononucleosis (sometimes referred to as "the kissing disease"), a cancer common in Africa known as Burkitt's lymphoma, and possibly chronic Epstein-Barr virus syndrome. Most of the time, however, it simply infects us without causing any illness; the majority of U.S. adults have antibodies to this virus, evidence that they have been infected with it some time in the past, whether or not they became sick. So while infectious diseases behave most clearly like "things," it is important to realize the role of your body in determining whether or not they produce illness and the role of your doctor in organizing the signs and symptoms of your illness into a disease.

For example, as we will see in the chapter on "Lime" disease, there has been considerable latitude in making diagnoses such as "Lyme disease." Some doctors would insist on isolating the spirochete associated with Lyme disease from the body; some would label as diseased those people who have certain symptoms of illness and show antibodies to the Lyme spirochete; some are content simply to find antibodies to the spirochete. Still other doctors diagnose Lyme disease on the basis of vague symptoms even when the antibodies cannot be found. The number of people who would be diagnosed as having Lyme disease will vary widely depending upon which definition is used.

The second type of disease is a described and recognizable combination of symptoms and signs. A migraine headache, which combines headache with stomach upset and sometimes with visual hallucinations, is an example of this type of disease. Here the role of the doctor in describing what constitutes a migraine headache is clear. However, few migraines actually fit neatly into this description, and doctors have the choice of either enlarging the description or finding a different term for those diseases that seem to have many things in common with a migraine but don't quite fit the criteria.

The third type of disease involves disorders of structure, while the fourth involves disorders of function; here we get into another type of trouble. Many of us have a variety of abnormalities in structure or function, but does this constitute a disorder? Take fibroid tumors of the uterus, for example. At least 25 percent of women have them, and while some fibroids are associated with heavy bleeding or other difficulties, many cause no problems at all. So are fibroids a disease or simply a variant of the normal female uterus?

WHAT'S NORMAL?

To complicate this last category of disease, physicians often don't know what normal is. When pathologists perform autopsies on people who have died, they often turn up "things" that were just sitting there, not causing any apparent problem and not discovered until the person died of something else. About 80 percent of all men above a certain age have some degree of cancer of the prostate, and about one-fourth of women consecutively autopsied in Denmark were found to have some degree of breast cancer. Nearly one-fourth of people autopsied will be found to have tumors of their pituitary gland. These tumors have been baptized *incidentalomas* because they were found "incidentally" at autopsy, apparently having caused no problem during the person's life.

While autopsies are performed too late for disease-mongers to benefit from their findings, some of the new imaging technologies can turn up all kinds of abnormalities about which no one quite knows what should be done. A woman sent for ultrasound examination of her pelvis may be told she has an "ovarian cyst," without the explanation that ovaries that are functioning normally produce cysts every month. Incidentalomas of the pituitary and adrenal glands are now found before autopsy in people who are undergoing scans for other reasons, and they sometimes lead to surgery. Many people, given the right tests, will be found to have gallstones that cause them no trouble at all—until their doctor convinces them to undergo surgery.

When people without any particular symptoms of gallbladder disease are screened by ultrasound, over 20 percent are found to have gallstones. Even if doctors consider removing the gallbladder in only those people who have gallstones *and* symptoms, the surgery won't relieve the symptoms of many of their patients; 35 percent of the population have symptoms of abdominal disease whether or not they have gallstones, so it's likely that in many persons who have both gallstones *and* symptoms the symptoms are not due to the presence of gallstones.

The problem is even more acute for older people, since less is known about what is "normal" in the elderly. According to a study reported in the *Journal of the American Medical Association* in 1991, when ultrasound examinations were given to residents of an older Jewish institution in Montreal, 80 percent of those over the age of 90 were found to have gallstones. "When do gallstones matter?" wrote Jack Ratner, M.D., chief author of the study. "Because many of these patients are studied by ultrasound, the finding of gallstones may lead to unjustifiable cholecystectomies [surgical removal of the gall bladder]."

Just how little medical science understands about the range of normality was shown by a recent Norwegian study reported in the *British Medical Journal*. People who have stomach complaints are often studied by means of a tube, known as an endoscope, that is put down into their stomach; doctors typically find that nine of ten have some abnormality, which they consider the cause of the symptoms. But the Norwegian doctors somehow persuaded people who had no complaints to undergo endoscopy (Norwegians have a reputation for stoicism), and they found that 90 percent of these seemingly normal volunteers also had some abnormality of their stomach lining, raising questions as to whether the symptoms were related to the abnormalities. "Only one in ten people," according to the editorial that accompanied the findings, "had an entirely normal upper GI [gastrointestinal] tract. . . . For the individual, a normal upper gut is one that does what is asked of it without complaint. For doctors and scientists, much more research stands between them and a working definition of normality."

One classic study done in the 1930s showed that perhaps doctors *need* to find a certain percentage of people abnormal and in need of treatment. The American Child Health Association surveyed 1000 children, all age 11, in New York City public schools. A total of 61 percent had already had their tonsils removed. When the remaining 39 percent were examined by a group of physicians, the doctors decided that 45 percent needed a tonsillectomy. When the children said not to need the operation were then examined by another group of physicians, 46 percent were judged to need tonsillectomy. When yet a third group of physicians examined the dwindling group of supposedly "healthy" children, they recommended the operation in about 45 percent. After three diagnostic passes, only 65 children, or 6.5 percent had not had a recommendation for tonsillectomy. "These subjects were not further examined because the supply of examining physicians ran out," commented Harry Bakwin, M.D., in the *New England Journal of Medicine*.

Bearing in mind the risks and hazards involved in most medical procedures, we can see the real danger of harming people by treating them for what is essentially a normal—and nonproblematic—condition. Until the late 1950s, doctors considered the enlarged thymus glands found in some infants as a disease, "status thymicolymphaticus," and treated them with irradiation. Eventually it was realized that the thymuses of people treated for this condition were actually normal, but the girls so irradiated faced an increased risk of breast cancer later in life and children of both sexes an increased risk of thyroid cancer.

OTHER SOURCES OF "DISEASE"

Three other phenomena deserve comment here, because they are often called diseases in America today.

The first is the "diseasing" of what are essentially risk factors for other diseases, such as high blood pressure and high cholesterol. Extremely high blood pressure might be considered a disease in itself, since it can cause the blood vessels in the brain to break, leading to stroke. But moderately raised blood pressure is more of a risk factor: It is associated with an increased *risk* of heart attack and stroke, but neither event is inevitable, and the likelihood of its happening depends heavily upon the presence of other risk factors. Similarly, a high cholesterol level is not a disease in itself, but the higher the cholesterol level, the more likely the person is to have a heart attack. (See Chapter 12 for a more detailed discussion of high blood pressure and cholesterol.)

While risk factors can be useful guides in medicine, the diseasing of them has led to lapses in medical logic. High blood pressure, for example, in both men and women is associated with an increased risk of stroke and heart attack; but blood pressure readings being equal, the risk is much less in women. In fact, several major studies have shown that women who have only slightly elevated blood pressure are *more* likely to die if they take drugs to reduce their blood pressure than those who are not treated.

After menopause, however, women are more likely to have high blood pressure than men of comparable age, leading some to proclaim that high blood pressure is therefore a bigger problem for women than for men. This leads doctors to treat the slightly raised blood pressure of an enormous number of women, even though there's no evidence to show that such treatment will benefit them by lowering the risk of heart attack or stroke: the treatment simply lowers their blood pressure, which in the absence of its link to other diseases is irrelevant. By considering high blood pressure a disease, the level of the numbers, rather than any consequence they might lead to, has become of primary importance.

"Disease is a rare event, and physicians have run out of diseases, but you never run out of risk factors," explains Rodney Jackson, M.D., a professor of epidemiology at the University of Auckland in New Zealand. "When you treat risk factors, you'll never be without a job."

The second phenomenon is the "medicalization" of life events, such as childbirth and menopause, converting these normal processes into diseases to be treated. As with treating risk factors, medicalization assures that no matter how many doctors, there will always be enough "disease" to keep them busy.

The third phenomenon, well documented by Stanton Peele in his book *Diseasing of America*, is the diseasing of addictions, starting with alcoholism but extending to drug addictions, codependency, and even love and sex addictions. The United States "has always been a leader in diseasing everything because, more than any other country, it has that kind of love with medicalization and the concept that we should be able to cure everything." Peele points out that in numerous other countries, such as Britain, "many find it less useful to call alcoholism a disease. It is not accidental that reimbursement of doctors [there] is not dependent on what is defined as a disease or not, whereas in the U.S. the reward structure is built on fitting as many things as possible into the doctor's bag."

The concept of "codependency" allows an even greater expansion of the number of people labeled sick, since there can be several codependents for every person with an addiction. As Marlon T. Gieser wrote in a letter to the *New York Times Book Review*, when families of substance abusers changed from 'victims' into 'sick codependents,' a new class of billable patients was created. "Family members who were once 'educated' as part of the patient's therapeutic program now receive their own psychiatric diagnoses, concurrent 'therapeutic' programs, and monthly statements geared to medical insurance reimbursement."

Ellen Goodman, writing in *Newsday*, pinpointed one thing wrong with many psychiatric diagnoses—and diagnoses in general—when she discussed Kitty Dukakis's chronicle of her addictions, *Now You Know*, and her often-repeated statement, "I'm Kitty Dukakis and I'm a drug addict and an alcoholic." Wrote Goodman:

> Hidden is the woman who is funny as well as intense, an enthusiastic gossip about life and love, a talker and a listener, passionate about her family, her politics, her projects. . . . What troubles me the most in this dutiful, serious, uncompromising effort at truth-telling is what the culture of addiction treatment seems to demand of the troubled in this era. Your whole identity. . . . Today Kitty Dukakis describes herself by her diagnoses. Drug addict. Alcoholic. Manic depressive. As one of many who have known her, I hope that behind that list are words without prescription pads—'compassionate' and 'strong'—just waiting to reappear.

Many people staunchly defend the idea of alcoholism as a disease: since we have already seen that there is no real agreement on what constitutes a disease, there's no real reason that alcoholism can't be one. Many people believe that considering alcoholism as a disease relieves its stigma, and they often claim that it should be no more stigmatized than diabetes, overlooking the fact that diabetics are often stigmatized because of the link of some forms of diabetes to overeating.

But when you attempt to ask people what they mean by the disease "alcoholism," things get murkier. Some people say they mean that there is a genetic susceptibility, which is defining it more like a risk factor.

When you ask people to define what constitutes alcoholism, things get even murkier. Some people say that if you ever desire an alcoholic beverage, that makes you an alcoholic. Some people say you're an alcoholic if you drink every day, while others would refine that to cover a certain quantity every day. Some doctors say you're alcoholic if you drink more than they—the doctors themselves—do. Some say you're alcoholic if your drinking interferes with your work, and some if your work interferes with your drinking.

Perhaps the most useful definition of alcoholism is this one: when your drinking causes, or will cause in the long run, more pain than pleasure. This, in fact, is near to what should be the definition of any disease: that point at which diagnosis and treatment are likely to improve our lives from what they would otherwise be, which, of course, can be a highly subjective judgment.

THE POLITICAL ASPECT OF DISEASE

While the diagnosis of disease is most useful when there is at least a chance that it will benefit individual patients, there are many others beside the patient who have a stake in the definition of disease. As Thomas S. Szasz, author of *The Myth of Mental Illness*, puts it:

> Who is helped and who is harmed by classifying a certain "condition"—be it paresis, paranoia or pathologic gambling— as a disease? What political values and social interests are advanced or retarded by classifying a certain person (e.g., someone who masturbates, malingers, or murders) as sick? . . . I should emphasize that all definitions are made of certain purposes, and that since different individuals and institutions have different interests, conflicts concerning the definitions—of disease or of any other concept or category with practical consequences—are likely to reflect their respective desires.

People agitate for or against enlarging the category of illness—for or against counting masturbation, unwanted pregnancy, smoking, rape, or murder as disease—because they desire or detest the consequences. Two of the most important consequences of the idea of mental illness are the deprivation of innocent persons of liberty, called "civil commitment," and the declaration of persons guilty of crimes as innocent, called a successful insanity defense. Indeed, it is precisely these interventions that make insanity an attractive idea to some people and an unattractive one to others.

While Dr. Szasz was talking about the diagnosis of mental illness, as I hope to show you in the following chapters, there is a political aspect to the diagnosis of physical disease, too.

Chapter 3

The Misuse of Diagnostic Tests

We are a testing culture: we test our urine for drugs, we test our sweat for lies.
—*New England Journal of Medicine*, July 23, 1987. Klemens B. Meyer and Stephen G. Pauker, vol. 314, no. 19.

The only two mammals to remove blood regularly from other mammals are vampire bats and humans.
—*New England Journal of Medicine*, 1986. vol. 314, no. 19.

One day while flipping through medical journals in the library, I came upon an article that at first puzzled, then horrified, me. A woman physician writing in the *British Medical Journal* recounted how during a pregnancy she had taken a test that showed antibody to the protozoa known as *Toxoplasma gondii* in her blood. Because of this, her doctor advised her to have an abortion. Here I was already a bit puzzled. I knew that if the infection known as toxoplasmosis *starts* during pregnancy it *may* (but doesn't always) damage the fetal nervous system. But simply finding antibody to *Toxoplasma gondii* in her blood could also mean that the woman had been infected before her pregnancy, in which case she had little to fear, at least from toxoplasmosis.

I continued reading. The woman aborted her pregnancy. Since the woman's antibody levels did not fall to zero, she finally went ahead and got pregnant again against medical advice. Here I was even more puzzled: once you are infected with *Toxoplasma gondii*, your antibody levels *never* fall to zero. Since by now she knew that her infection had preceded the pregnancy, there was no reason in the world, at least concerning toxoplasmosis, that a doctor should advise against becoming pregnant. In France, for example, all women of childbearing age are routinely screened for antibody to *Toxoplasma gondii*; those who test positive are told that they can get pregnant without fear because once you've had toxoplasmosis (as evidenced by the antibodies), you probably won't get it again.

The woman's story continued. Her obstetrician decided to treat the fetus in utero, killing it in the process. An analysis showed that it was not, in fact, infected with *Toxoplasma gondii*, something anyone who knew anything about toxoplasmosis would have known. The story was a very poignant one about grieving for her dead fetus, whom she named Adam. Only in the end did the woman acknowledge that the treatment was probably unnecessary.

By this time I was livid. The story of Adam was a vivid example of the human tragedies that can result from using a diagnostic test without having a clue as to what the results mean.

The 5 to 10 billion medical tests ordered in the United States every year cost as much as $27 billion, about 6 percent of the nation's health care budget and as much as the combined spending on drugs and medical supplies. Diagnostic procedures such as endoscopies, lab tests, and imaging procedures accounted for about 30 percent of the Medicare expenditures in 1989. Many of these tests are quite useful and lead to improved diagnosis and treatment. But Robert H. Brook, a professor of medicine at the University of California at Los Angeles, says that "at least a third if not more than half of what we do is of no benefit or of such marginal benefit that I think we could reach agreement in society that insurance should not pay for it."

Most people seem to regard tests as more valid, more important, and less harmful than they really are. On the individual level they are the American placebo, and at the social level people seem to regard testing as a solution in itself, without asking what they are going to do with the results. If diseasing something is a way of passing the buck, testing is regarded as magic. When, for example, a child died of lead poisoning in Michigan, there was a call for screening for lead poisoning. But when you read the circumstances, you found that the child was homeless, living in an abandoned building. Calling for blood testing was obviously easier than calling for a policy of providing safe and low-cost shelter for the poor, but who can doubt which policy would really benefit such children more? While posters around New York are calling for people to take an AIDS test, only a minority of those infected have money or health insurance to pay for treatment, and in the absence of a significant public commitment, coming in for AIDS testing will have done nothing to benefit these individuals. "Those who test positive and lack health insurance may find themselves in a three-month line just to see a doctor, let alone gain access to costly life-prolonging therapies," wrote Erik Eckholm in the *New York Times.*

THE DOWNSIDE OF TESTING

Calls for testing rarely acknowledge that there is a considerable downside to testing that includes but goes beyond the dollar cost. This view of tests and screening as magic overlooks the following realities:

- *Diagnostic testing is largely unregulated, even at the elementary level of ensuring that equipment is accurate and that trained people are reading the test results under optimal conditions.*
- *Even tests performed by well-trained people with standardized equipment often don't give good answers to the question, Does this person have a particular disease or not? Sometimes they don't even help answer that question.*
- *A positive test for a condition you are unlikely to have is more likely to be a false positive than a true positive.*
- *Even good tests, performed under good conditions, don't always lead to improved therapy, and they can take a significant toll in side effects.*

- *Diagnostic testing is largely unregulated.* Basically, regulation doesn't exist and, to a certain extent, won't for a long time because there is currently so much disagreement about testing. Some states partially regulate laboratories and equipment, but until now there has been little regulation at the federal level. A law, the Clinical Laboratory Improvement Amendments, was passed in 1988 but wasn't implemented for four years because, according to Gail R. Wilensky, head of the Federal Health Care Financing Administration, "the statute assumed a consensus in the scientific community about the complexity and riskiness of lab tests that simply does not exist."

The amendments are scheduled to take effect September 1, 1992, but the standards will be phased in over the next two years, possibly longer. These are minimum standards and could eliminate conditions where doctors' wives and secretaries read the results of Pap smears. They cannot, however, deal with the fact that there is substantial disagreement among pathologists and other testers themselves.

• *Even tests performed by well-trained people with standardized equipment give highly variable results.* Part of this variability is due to the fact that the human body varies from moment to moment, from day to day, and from year to year. Your blood pressure can vary widely, for example, depending upon whether it's being taken by a doctor or a nurse, a man or a woman, whether you're sitting or standing and for how long, whether it's morning, afternoon, or evening, and whether you're nervous. Cholesterol readings also vary according to a number of factors, including emotional ones, as do tests of blood glucose and platelet reactivity. "If a specimen is split and analyzed by two laboratories," wrote Peter Rasmussen, M.D., of the University of Maryland School of Medicine, "the two measurements of the same analyte will almost always differ, and sometimes the difference may be substantial. . . . Results for enzymes are particularly variable, as are those for cholesterol, triglycerides, high-density lipoprotein (HDL) cholesterol, and ammonia. Even the total white blood cell count may vary considerably."

Pathologists can also differ on their judgment of whether a tissue is benign or malignant. While laymen assume that a tumor either is or is not cancer, in reality many tumors are somewhere in between. This is particularly true for endometrial carcinoma, the cancer of the inner lining of the uterus. One pathologist, for example, told me that she had trained at Stanford, which tends to be conservative: "I would tend to label hyperplasia (benign proliferation of cells) what others here might call carcinoma (cancerous proliferation of cells)." Another, J. Donald Woodruff, M.D., professor of gynecologic pathology at Johns Hopkins University School of Medicine, told a session of the 1986 meeting of the American College of Obstetricians and Gynecologists that about one-third of the cases of diagnosed endometrial cancer are not cancer but hyperplasia. While regulation of labs might make certain that trained pathologists were reading the results, it cannot really handle the fact that pathologists trained at Stanford may disagree with those trained at Harvard.

Sometimes supposedly well trained people will develop a "test" that no one else seems able to use. In 1984, the chief of cytopathology at a southern medical school started diagnosing cancer by staining cells obtained by biopsies with a stain called B72.3. According to an episode on the television program "20/20," patient Betty Eldreth was told, on the basis of the stain, that her breast cancer had spread to her rib, for which she underwent weeks of radiation therapy that has left her arm permanently swollen. She was also told that a mass in her abdomen was cancerous; when the mass was removed, it was found not to be cancerous, which was when doctors began to suspect that something was wrong. Another physician at the same university, Dr. Ken McCarty, says that the B72.3 test was used on 5,000 patients, probably misdiagnosing cancer one-third of the time.

Considering the amount of difference among pathologists, who have trained for years to interpret cancer slides, imagine what the differences are among doctors untrained in interpreting tests and trying to incorporate new ones into their practices. Often they may not actually test what they claim to be testing. Even when they do, there's little information on whether the benefits of performing the tests outweigh the costs and risks. A survey by the American College of Chest Physicians found the tests most commonly used for acute myocardial infarction (MI) (heart attack) were exercise test (52 percent), echocardiography (48 percent), and Holter monitoring (46 percent). "What evidence do we have that any of these procedures in fact improves the outlook for the patient with an acute MI?" commented Dr. James Dalen, then-chairman of the Department of Medicine at the University of Massachusetts Medical School. "I know of no evidence. It's clear that we use a double standard. For drugs we have to have a randomized clinical trial. But for a diagnostic test, someone describes it, and we buy it and we do it."

Testing for Thoracic Outlet Syndrome

Consider a test described in the *New England Journal of Medicine* in 1972 and used for many years afterward to identify a condition known as "thoracic outlet syndrome." Classic thoracic outlet syndrome, in which the arm becomes weak and atrophies, can occur in people who have an occluded blood vessel, and this condition is relatively easy to diagnose. Very rarely, a condition known as "neurogenic" thoracic outlet syndrome results when an extra rib rubs against the ulnar nerve, which runs from the spinal cord to the ring and little fingers. This condition, too, is easy to identify: all the doctor has to do is to see the extra rib on the X ray, although most people with these extra ribs do not have symptoms. But some doctors began extrapolating from these relatively rare patients with extra ribs to a much wider group of patients who had vague symptoms in their arms similar to those seen in some people with extra ribs. They reasoned that perhaps one of the normal ribs was irritating the ulnar nerve, and they began removing normal ribs.

But since weakness in the arm is a fairly subjective symptom, this lesser degree of thoracic outlet syndrome was difficult to identify, and many patients who had a rib removed to treat their "thoracic outlet syndrome" continued to have symptoms. The test described in the *New England Journal* was an attempt to identify those patients who might benefit from rib removal.

Twelve years after the test was first described, Drs. Asa J. Wilbourn and Richard J. Lederman of the Cleveland Clinic Foundation wrote to the *New England Journal*, noting that in their hands the test had not worked very well as a way to identify patients who would benefit from surgery. More alarmingly, however, they alleged that the diagram published with the original article couldn't be a real test result. The journal's editor referred the letter to the original authors, and the authors admitted they hadn't noticed that the diagram, which had been supplied by somebody else, couldn't really be what they said it was. Dr. Arnold Relman wrote a scathing editorial pointing out that not only had the authors not carried out the nerve conduction tests themselves, but they were not familiar enough with the test itself to recognize that the people who had performed it had given them a test result that had been manipulated to make it appear better for publication. "When authors discuss and advocate the clinical use of a diagnostic procedure," he wrote, "and when they publish illustrations of its applications in specific patients, I think they ought to know something about the procedure itself."

While this was a particularly egregious example of how little widely used diagnostic tests are monitored, many other tests fall down when subjected to close scrutiny of whether they test what they claim they are testing. The two classic measures of how well a test measures what it is supposed to are known as sensitivity and specificity. Sensitivity is a measure of how well the test picks up people who really have the disease (true positives), and specificity measures how many people the tests say don't have the disease really do not (true negatives). In both cases, the higher the number the better. People who have the disease but test negative are known as false negatives, and those who don't have the disease but give a positive test are known as false positives. A test is a good one when there are few false positives or false negatives.

Diagnosing the "Mouth Breather"

Consider the diagnosis of "mouth breathing." This is supposed to mean that a child breathes mostly through the mouth, often because the adenoids are encroaching on the nasal passages. While adenoids shrink with age, the parents may be told that children who breathe through the mouth will develop an elongated lower face. Parents are also told that this "facial deformity" could jeopardize the results of orthodontic work. Orthodontists therefore try to identify mouth breathers and urge their parents to have the condition corrected, often by having their adenoids removed.

Orthodontists will ask the mother if the child breathes through the mouth, explains Peter Vig, D.D.S., a professor of orthodontics at the University of Pittsburgh, and since nearly all children under the age of ten or so walk around with their lips apart, the mother may say yes, leading to a series of tests that purportedly identify a large number of mouth breathers for whom surgery is recommended. "A surprisingly large number of clinicians in this country now recommend surgical intervention or other forms of nonorthodontic treatment directed at 'improving' nasal airway function," according to Dr. Vig. In at least one major American university in recent years several hundred operations, such as adenoidectomy, reduction of the turbinate bones that project into the nose, and corrections of deviated septa, were performed on children between one and five years of age at the recommendation of orthodontists. Dr. Vig questioned whether, in fact, mouth breathing really led to deformity. Even more fundamentally, he questioned whether anyone really knew what a "mouth breather" was.

Two methods are commonly used to test for "mouth breathing," he explains. One is an X ray of the skull profile known as the cephalogram, which allows calculation of the size of the air passages in the nose and pharynx. If this size is below a certain critical value, it is assumed that the person has to be a "mouth breather" simply because the nasal airway seems to be constricted. The other method is a test of the air flow through the nose, called rhinomanometry, where a given value of resistance is often considered evidence that the person breathes through the mouth. Neither method, however, really measures that proportion of breathing occurring through the nose and that proportion through the mouth. Dr. Vig also found that nobody seemed to be able to define what proportion of air flow through the mouth was needed to qualify for the diagnosis of "mouth breather."

Dr. Vig and his associates decided that knowing this proportion was necessary to diagnose "mouth breathing" properly. He and his associates developed a technique they baptized "SNORT" (simultaneous nasal and oral respirometric technique), which, in fact, measured the proportion of breathing through the nose and the proportion through the mouth. Comparing the cephalogram and rhinomanometry with SNORT, he found that the former— the two most commonly used diagnostic tests—were no better than flipping a coin in determining who was really a mouth breather. For example, one of the measures calculated from the cephalogram, used to identify how much of the breathing space is being occupied by the adenoids, had a sensitivity of 18.2, meaning that it picked up only one-fifth of true mouth breathers, and a specificity of 66.6, meaning that of the people it diagnosed as not being mouth breathers, only two-thirds really weren't. Second, he found that 90 percent of people do most of their breathing through their noses. Third, he found that even if someone did 100 percent of their breathing through the mouth, it didn't necessarily make much difference.

In nine years of performing SNORT tests, says Dr. Vig, he has found only three teenagers who breathed totally through their mouths, and they seemed perfectly normal. "They looked just like everyone else: there was nothing wrong with their facial features."

Dr. Vig acknowledges that there may be reasons to treat mouth breathers, for example, if their mouth breathing is bothering them or causing troublesome symptoms. But simply to use tests to identify mouth breathers—when the tests are no better than flipping a coin, and the significance of mouth breathing remains to be determined—should, he believes, be stopped.

He also believes that the fact that orthodontists refer their patients to ear, nose, and throat surgeons actually *increases* the chances that patients will have something done to them, a belief that goes against conventional wisdom that overuse is more a problem when patients go directly to surgeons, who then operate on them. When an orthodontist tells an ear, nose, and throat (ENT) surgeon that he wants a child evaluated for mouth breathing in order to prevent facial deformity, the ENT surgeon simply assumes that the orthodontist knows what he is talking about. The ENT surgeon may not feel that the adenoids are causing any particular problem, but he or she will remove them anyway, since the orthodontist has assured him or her that the operation is necessary.

Diagnosing on the Curve

Still another problem with tests in which there is a spectrum of values (such as blood counts) is that in some cases people just take the top 2.5 percent and the bottom 2.5 percent and label them as being outside the normal range. In other words, a certain percentage of the population is defined as abnormal simply be-cause they are at the outer ends of normality. It's a bit like grading on the curve: the testers have decided that *somebody* has to be abnormal. This doesn't necessarily mean, however, that they have any condition that's going to cause them problems. Because "normal" has often been defined for a specific reference group—say, young, white men, often those who happened to be working in a hospital and therefore available—women, blacks, or older people may, in fact, have a probability greater than 5 per-cent of falling outside these normal limits, yet they may not be "sick."

So, even if you're healthy, having one test done still gives you a 1-in-20 chance of being given a label that could be interpreted as meaning that you are sick. If you have 20 tests done, which is not uncommon in a biochemical profile, there's a 64 percent chance that one test will be abnormal EVEN IF YOU'RE HEALTHY. If you have 100 tests done, the chance of one test's being abnormal is 99.4 percent!

• *A positive test for a condition you are unlikely to have is more likely to be a false positive than a true positive.* At first glance this seems hard to believe, but it's really simple arithmetic and is known as Baye's rule or Baye's theorem after the eighteenth-century English clergyman Samuel Bayes. Baye's theorem is based on the fact that even a small percentage of false positives—say, 1 percent—multiplied by the large numbers of people who don't have the disease, will produce a significant number of false positives. If the disease is uncommon, the number of false positives will probably be higher than the number of people who really have the disease.

False Positives and the AIDS Virus

Suppose, for example, that in a particular test for the HIV or AIDS virus, of every ten positives nine will be true positives and one will be a false positive. This is known as a specificity of .90 and is pretty good as tests go.

But suppose that 1 percent of the residents of New Hampshire, which has a population of about 1 million, really are infected with the AIDS virus, and you decide to test all 1 million residents. If the test is 100 percent sensitive, you may pick up all the 10,000 true positives (1 percent of 1 million), but you'll also pick up 10 percent of the 990,000 people who don't have the virus as false positives, meaning that you have 99,000 false positives, nearly ten times as many people as are truly positive. This means that for every true case of HIV positivity identified—and one might argue that knowing this has advantages—there will be ten people who risk losing their jobs, losing health insurance, or even commit suicide because of the false diagnosis.

Supposedly the tests done by a good lab are more accurate. But a study in 1987 by the Office of Technology Assessment, reported in *U. S. News & World Report*, found that for groups at low risk of AIDS, 9-in-10 positive findings were false positives. The main reason, the study said, was that many labs perform the Western blot—the second of two tests routinely used to detect AIDS infection—very poorly. Because at that time some 7 percent of the U.S. population had already gotten the test, hundreds and possibly thousands of people believe they have the virus when they don't.

Even if the test is much more specific, with a false positive rate of 0.5 percent instead of 10 percent, it will still find more false positives than true positives if the incidence of disease is low enough. Drs. Klemens B. Meyer and Stephen G. Parker, writing in the *New England Journal of Medicine*, pointed out that if only 0.01 percent of the population really are infected with the AIDS virus, as was found a few years ago for the population of women blood donors, even a test that's 99.5 percent specific will still identify 50 women as false positives for every woman who is really infected. "If laws are to link our fates to test results," Drs. Meyer and Parker wrote, "should not due process be brought to the benches where those tests are performed?"

A few years after their article was published, I asked Dr. Meyer how the real sensitivity and specificity of the AIDS test compared to their theoretical calculations. Dr. Meyer responded that while studies had been performed showing that the sensitivity and specificity of the tests were quite good in theory, sometimes they were not as good as performed in practice. A pregnant woman in the Boston area had recently been told her AIDS test was positive, for example, because the doctor wasn't skilled in interpreting the results.

"As a practicing physician, I don't know what quality controls are in place for the performance of this test," he said. "I don't know enough to counsel patients—and I probably know more than most doctors, having written a paper about precisely this subject." Dr. Meyer said that while he was now working in an area other than that of AIDS testing, he did "read what comes across my desk on the subject." Data on the sensitivity and specificity of the AIDS test are not readily made available to practicing physicians. "And that's also true of all the other tests I order," he said.

Advocates of testing will argue that in a good testing program people would be counseled and told that in fact their results might be false positives. But while David Morgan, who had to undergo an HIV test for insurance purposes in England (the insurance company demanded a test because Morgan had once requested a test for HIV on his own, which appeared to the insurance company as suspicious behavior), was told that he would be counseled, he found the counseling lacking, to say the least. "As the general practitioner prepared to take a sample, I said that the advice sheet I had received mentioned counselling before I consented to the test," Morgan wrote in the *British Medical Journal.* "He glanced at the sheet and remarked that it was not necessary to go through all that, adding, 'Anyway, you know about AIDS, don't you? It's a bloody disaster. If you've got it you're dead.' Nothing more was said about either the clinical aspects of AIDS or the social implications of being tested."

AIDS, of course, is a particularly bad-case scenario, and it is complicated by the fact that there are serious public health implications: some people might judge trying to prevent the spread of the virus important enough to justify the thousands of lives of healthy people that will be sacrificed in a testing program (although whether testing will really help keep the virus from spreading isn't known). But nearly all tests can cause emotional turmoil, as well as an inability to get jobs or health insurance.

Furthermore, few tests are as specific as even 90 percent. Dr. Richard Wernick, of the Oregon Health Sciences University in Portland, in a recent article in *Geriatrics* showed how the rules pertained to a hypothetical 70-year-old woman with stiffness and knobby hands, who ends up testing positive for both the rheumatoid factor, used in the diagnosis of rheumatoid arthritis, and ANA, one of the tests for systemic lupus erythematosus, an autoimmune disease with many symptoms similar to those of rheumatoid arthritis. If the doctor interprets the positive test for rheumatoid arthritis as meaning that this woman has the disease, he will be incorrect 93 percent of the time, Dr. Wernick points out. If he interprets the positive ANA test as meaning the woman has lupus, he will be incorrect over 99 percent of the time, with the woman having only a 0.7 percent chance of really having lupus.

The willy-nilly use of tests goes beyond turning up false positives. It can turn up people who really have some degree of abnormality, but since the abnormality is less than that which doctors have any experience in treating, they don't really know if people will be better off with treatment than without. Hyperparathyroidism, overactivity of the parathyroid gland, used to be diagnosed only in those patients who had symptoms such as nervousness, and it was treated by removing the parathyroid glands. But now, with screening, the incidence of patients who get the label of hyperparathyroidism has jumped tenfold, and doctors don't know how to treat them. Will they really be better off having this chemical abnormality corrected, or will more die and have complications from the surgery itself than will be helped?

• *Even good tests, performed under good conditions, don't always lead to improved therapy, and they can take a significant toll in side effects.* It's of course not very useful to order a test when the results, whatever they are, are not in any way going to change the treatment. A pregnant woman opposed to abortion who undergoes amniocentesis to detect a birth defect for which the only "treatment" is abortion might be the classic case of this. One might argue that she wants to know whether she's going to have an abnormal child so she can prepare for it psychologically, but when the only treatment possible is unacceptable, she is probably better off not knowing. Since amniocentesis itself can cause abortion, and perhaps even minor forms of birth defects, the risk here would really seem to be greater than the benefit.

Electronic monitoring of the fetal heart rate while a pregnant woman is in labor has never been shown to produce healthier babies, even though it leads to a higher rate of cesarean sections. In fact, one study reported by Lawrence Altman in the New York Times found that babies monitored electronically had three times the rate of cerebral palsy as babies monitored with a stethoscope.

The FDA has recently approved a device for monitoring uterine activity at home, which is being marketed to pregnant women as a way to prevent premature births. The system costs over $5,000 per patient, yet while there is evidence that it can help detect certain signs and symptoms of preterm labor, there's no evidence that it can prevent premature births. The overwhelming majority of premature babies, in fact, are born to poor women with little or no neonatal care, and if the nation wants to do something about preventing prematurity, efforts should be directed to these women, not those who can invest $5,000.

But the person at the FDA responsible for approving the device, Lillian Yin, Ph.D., presented the FDA's position that approval didn't necessarily mean that the device would help anyone, simply that it could detect what it claimed to detect, uterine contractions. "Requiring proof that the device prevents premature births as a condition of marketing approval would impose a therapeutic outcome as the end point for a monitoring device," Dr. Yin wrote in the New England Journal of Medicine. Moreover, she said, to base its approval on the fact that it was actually able to prevent premature labor, "the FDA would first need to be certain that there was a successful treatment for the disease or condition being diagnosed. Such a regulatory position would be detrimental to public health."

While taking such a limited view of regulation may be justified, the next time anyone says that something is FDA-approved you should remember that this doesn't necessarily mean that it offers any benefit.

Tests have all kinds of side effects. Betty Eldreth, who underwent weeks of unnecessary radiation therapy and ungrounded surgery, suffered from the effect of a test that itself hadn't been adequately tested, and Adam's mother, who was advised incorrectly to have an abortion and whose second fetus was killed in utero, suffered from a test that the doctor knew how to perform but not to interpret. Even interpretable and tested tests, however, don't always help. Dr. Barbara Thomas, director of the Guildford breast screening project in England, pointed out that "every cancer detected means that a woman has the label, the misery, and the decreased quality of life. The gain is an extension of life, but that is only achieved for a third of patients."

In a perfect world tests would not be performed unless there was at least a reasonable chance that they might benefit the patient. But just as the considerable leeway in deciding whether to call something a disease or not can give an opening to people who profit from calling it a disease, the decision to perform a test, or at what point to consider the results abnormal, can also be manipulated to give results not necessarily based on benefit to the patient. Many people make money from tests, and tests are a major way that well people become convinced that they are really sick. It's worthwhile examining just who has an interest in getting you tested as the first step to convincing you that you're sick.

Chapter 4

The Players and the Payers

He understood that if you don't get into the business of doing early diagnosis, you run the risk of not getting the referrals that will fill up your beds and preserve your market share.
—The M.D. Who Would Be a Tycoon, *New York Times Magazine*, September 25, 1988.

Remember when you used to play the game of "gossip" as a child? A group would sit around in a circle, and one child would whisper something to the next, who would whisper the same thing to the next, and so on around the circle. Finally, the last child would compare what he or she had heard, which was usually something like "GMnnnnnnn" at that point, to what the first child had said. The message had gotten distorted, usually to the point that it no longer made any sense.

Messages are also distorted in the communication of medical information. There is, however, a dramatic difference between the game of gossip and the communication of medical information: while in the case of gossip the message becomes totally incomprehensible, in the case of medical information the message *appears* to make sense. But at each stage it has undergone a transformation that tends to simplify the reality. In most cases, the simplification has altered the message so that the disease sounds more serious than it really is, and the side effects of the diagnosis and treatment sound less significant than they really are. In other words, you no longer have the information you need

53

to make an informed choice on the issue: are the benefits of diagnosis and treatment greater than the risks?

This is because nearly everyone along the way—from the researchers who do the study to the medical journalists who write the articles you read, from the doctors who diagnose you to the hospitals to which they admit you, and the drug companies that provide your treatment—has an interest in convincing you that a given disease is widespread and serious. Some diseases are indeed widespread, some are quite serious, and a few are both. But it's worth keeping in mind that the life expectancy in most developed countries today is fairly good, at around 75 years for men and 80 for women, and that the type of medicine practiced in each of these countries differs quite dramatically, making it unlikely that most medical interventions play a major role in life expectancy. In other words, most people are "built" rather healthy, and if they live in an environment at least as benign as that of North America and Western Europe, their bodies can usually take pretty good care of themselves even without doctors. This is not to say that medicine can never prolong life or add to its quality, but it does mean that a healthy skepticism is called for when a medical test or intervention is prescribed.

The health field in general has been characterized by rapid growth in the past 20 years, with an increase in the number of doctors, for-profit hospitals, medical writers, drug promoters, and indeed almost everyone with a role. If the amount of "disease" in the community were finite, this would unquestionably be beneficial, with providers competing with each other to treat patients at the least possible cost and treating them as politely as possible so that they would keep coming back. But since disease is such a fluid and political concept, the providers can essentially create their own demand by broadening the definitions of diseases in such a way as to include the greatest number of people, and by spinning out new diseases.

Let us look at the each of the various groups in detail.

MEDICAL RESEARCHERS

Many medical researchers are the first to admit that what they do has a limited application in the short term. But medical researchers need funding in order to carry out their studies, and to do this, they must convince someone, usually either the government or a drug company, to give them money.

This means that, if they are seeking money from a government source, they must show that their research will be applicable as soon as possible. This probably accounts for the numerous stories, like the following, that constantly emanate from universities: "Early Detection of Alzheimer's May Be Only a Breath Away," says a Purdue University News Release, 1990. Not emphasized, of course, is that such a test must itself be tested against time: Do the patients who test positive on the test really develop Alzheimer's, and do the ones who test negative not get this disease? Perhaps more importantly, do you really want to know you are going to get Alzheimer's disease, when there's no effective prevention or treatment? The test may eventually prove useful to researchers and may ultimately benefit patients, but not until a prevention or cure is developed, and it could cause considerable mischief in the meantime. Yet the news article presents the item as an unmitigated good. "You can't overlook the role of investigator ego," points out Theodore L. Goodfriend, M.D., of the Departments of Pharmacology and Medicine, University of Wisconsin Medical School in Madison. "A researcher wants to believe what he's doing is important, and if he can't convince others he won't get promoted, he won't get funded, and he won't be able to go home with a sense of satisfaction."

Much medical research these days is funded by the pharmaceutical industry, and here there is always a certain amount of pressure to find results that will be favorable to the drug the company sells. Richard A. Davidson, M.D., an associate professor in the Department of Medicine at the University of Florida in Gainesville, found that studies supported by pharmaceutical companies were much more likely to find new therapies superior to old than were studies that apparently didn't receive funds from the pharmaceutical industry. In no case was a therapeutic agent manufactured by the sponsoring company found to be inferior to an alternative product manufactured by another company. If a drug company can see no potential benefit, it quite reasonably will not fund a study in the first place. The role of aspirin in preventing heart attacks was suspected as far back as the late 1940s, but well-controlled studies weren't done until recently.

According to Lawrence K. Altman, writing in the *New York Times*, "Because the patent on aspirin had long expired, experts say that drug companies had less incentive to push research on its benefits than they would on a new drug that they could have sold at a much higher price."

When a researcher completes a study, it becomes subject to what is known as publication bias. This means that if the results turn out not to show anything—for example, if they show that a treatment is of no benefit—the researchers will probably not submit them for publication. "The most serious potential consequence of this bias," wrote Philippa J. Easterbrook and her coworkers from the Johns Hopkins University School of Medicine in the *Lancet*, "would be an overestimate of treatment effects or risk-factor associations in published work."

Even if the researchers do submit the study, it may be less likely to be published. According to Samuel Shapiro, of the Boston University School of Medicine, "There is a strong tendency for editors to favor publishing positive rather than negative results, because negative findings are seldom novel. . . . The net effect of editorial policy is that there exists today a substantial selection bias in favor of the publication of positive results in medical journals." The supposed self-correcting mechanisms of science, where bad studies will eventually disappear because someone proves them wrong, don't always work as they are supposed to, either: Dr. Shapiro cites a study he and his coworkers undertook in response to a published "positive result". When Dr. Shapiro and his coworkers repeated the experiment and got a negative result instead of the positive one that had been published, they submitted it to the same journal. The editor did not question the validity of the study, but declined to publish the negative result, suggesting that the authors send it to another journal, and later suggesting that they write a Letter to the Editor. Dr. Shapiro and his coworkers found this unacceptable: "If an editorial decision is made to publish a positive finding, that decision carries with it the subsequent responsibility to publish the negative one."

In 1986, two researchers from the same team submitted two different papers to the *New England Journal of Medicine*. One of the papers, whose chief author was Dr. Charles D. Bluestone, claimed that treatment with the antibiotic amoxicillin reduced the severity of middle-ear infections. Dr. Bluestone had received approximately $260,000 in personal honoraria between 1983 and 1988, and $3.5 million in grants to his unit had been paid by pharmaceutical companies. Another paper, by a member of Dr. Bluestone's team, using a different analysis of the same data, found that the antibiotic was not effective. Only the paper claiming that the antibiotic was effective was initially published; the second paper was finally published by the *Journal of the American Medical Association* five years later. The second paper was returned by the *New England Journal of Medicine* with the comment: "The important question . . . is not whose interpretation is correct . . . but rather who has the right to publish." In the meantime, the author of the dissenting report was censured by his institution, the University of Pittsburgh, in reports that, according to the editor of the *Journal of the American Medical Association*, "read as if drawn up by the prosecution." While this case was complicated and the reason the one article was chosen wasn't necessarily that it was favorable to the antibiotic, the fact that the dissenting paper wasn't published for five years meant that antibiotic treatment of this condition appeared more favorable than it probably really was for that period of time.

A special type of publication should be mentioned here: the supplement to a regular medical journal. Such supplements are often totally supported by one drug company, and the articles in them often escape the normal review process used to decide whether a piece of work qualifies for publication in the regular pages of the journal. Yet people citing such studies often do not differentiate between these articles and those that appeared in the regular journal.

Publication bias has become particularly important now that many statisticians are doing *meta-analyses*, or analyses that lump together several studies that may have given contradictory results and so attempt to achieve a clear answer from them. If the statisticians analyze only published studies, they are likely to come up with the overestimate mentioned above. Since meta-analyses seem to carry a greater importance than single studies, their pronouncements could carry more weight than they really should. While Thomas Pickering, M.D., a professor of medicine at New York Hospital, notes that a proper meta-analysis should include unpublished data, "in practice this is practically never done."

Once a study is published, it becomes susceptible to what I will call *dissemination bias*. This means that if it meets the needs of any of the various players, they will see that it gets called to the attention of the press and of prescribing doctors. This is very important, since no journalist or doctor, no matter how dedicated, can keep up with more than a few journals. If a study supports a company's bottom line, the company will probably call it to the attention of doctors and medical journalists by, for example, holding a press conference followed by an elaborate lunch over which journalists can talk with the people who did the study. If the study is neutral or negative as far as the company's interest is concerned, it's up to the journalists to find it themselves.

MEDICAL WRITERS

Here I'm dealing with my own profession, and I have to cringe a bit at the comments of Jonathan Cole of Columbia University: "Those reporting on health risks do not, we assume, purposely distort facts, but their lack of knowledge of elementary statistics and probability and the basic analytic techniques of the sciences and social sciences almost always prevents them from getting it right."

What's interesting here, however, is that the more a medical writer learns about statistics and the more one's vision of medicine changes from black and white to various shades of gray, the harder it is to convince editors that you have a story. Editors like stories that at least have overtones of battles between good and evil: good patient against bad disease, good doctor against bad disease, good patient against bad doctor, and so on. They sometimes have little patience with the more complex realities: for example, this is a good drug for a few patients, but when overused, it causes an unacceptably high rate of complications. Since medical research really doesn't understand all that much about the human body and each medical study is a little like one of the blind men trying to figure out the nature of the elephant from only the trunk or tail or back, medical writers often find themselves writing contradictory stories from one day to the next. Yesterday's miracle drug becomes today's bad drug, and the story yesterday about people taking so many antibiotics that their germs are becoming resistant is forgotten in today's advice to take antibiotics to prevent Lyme disease.

The above problems result from deep-seated tendencies of American culture to see life as a battle of good against evil, to have a short memory, and to fail to attempt to resolve contradictions. There are also values more specific to the culture of journalism and values forced upon the publication by whoever is picking up the tab. All tend to bend medical stories in the same direction: to make diseases sound more widespread and serious than they really are and to minimize the side effects of treatment— at least until the side effects themselves become the story.

The culture of journalism has an interest in making a disease sound as serious and as widespread as possible; it simply makes a better story, one that will make the front page and the journalist's career. William Burrows, director of the Science and Environmental Reporting Program at New York University, says that journalists in general "always go with the worst possible case. If the Associated Press story reports that 50 people died in an airplane crash, and the United Press International story says 52, most papers will go with the figure of 52." Diseases that affect only a few people are simply not news material unless they can be used to illustrate some more common problem of health care. If a disease cannot be made to sound serious, many editors will use that favored question of editors: "So what?" The editors, of course, may well have a point in questioning whether a story should be run at all if not that many people are affected, and none that seriously.

The problem is that medical writers like to get their stories in, so they are under some pressure to hype the disease. Headlines, which are often all that many people read, tend to oversimplify even more. One of my favorites is one that appeared over an article in the *New York Times* pointing out that 80 percent of U.S. men had a cholesterol level greater than 180; the headline became "80 percent of U.S. males are at risk for premature death."

Besides the distortions that arise from the desire to make the disease seem as widespread and serious as possible is the fact that medical reporters decide which scientific papers will be reported by the extremely subjective criteria of which will make a "good story." What is somewhat frightening is that not only the lay public, but also the scientific community, will thus be directed to certain studies and away from others. David P. Phillips, Ph.D., and his coworkers at the University of California at San Diego, found that if a study from the *New England Journal of Medicine* is reported in the *New York Times*, it is more likely to be subsequently cited in the scientific literature than those studies not judged to be "good stories." It wasn't just that the reporters and the scientists were reaching the same conclusions independently: the *New England Journal* stories that made the *Times* when workers there were on strike, and the paper was therefore reaching very few people, were not more likely to be cited. The reporter's news judgment was therefore determining which medical knowledge got disseminated to the scientific community.

Still another way that journalists fall into the role of disease mongering is that they are afraid of reassuring people, since someone, inevitably, will run into complications, and the press, like other players, feel they will be judged more harshly for their sins of omission than for their sins of commission. If you tell someone to see a doctor because of a cold, and if the doctor prescribes penicillin and the patient dies of an allergic reaction, the journalist can always pass the buck to the doctor, who after all shouldn't have prescribed penicillin for just a cold. But if the journalist states that you don't have to see a doctor when you have a cold, and the patient really doesn't have a cold but has pneumonia, the journalist could conceivably be blamed. When I wrote an article for the *New York Mycological Society Newsletter* telling people that Lyme disease was curable and not as widespread as generally believed, and that perhaps we shouldn't worry about it all that much, another medical journalist thought I was being irresponsible. People shouldn't be reassured, he opined, because then they might not take precautions.

The same incentives apply to book writers, only more so. People will still buy newspapers even if they're not interested in the subject of all the stories, but few people will pay $20 for a book unless they're strongly convinced that it's of practical value to them. I had trouble selling the idea of my first book, *How to Avoid a Hysterectomy*, even though I was able to point out quite honestly that about one-third of American women had hysterectomies and the big wave of the baby-boom population was at the age where these women would be faced with the decision.

This was still not enough; one editor said that because so many women had already had hysterectomies, the population I could sell to would be too small.

The financial pressures on magazines are somewhat more complex. Here the disease must be serious and widespread, but there must also be a cure for it. The editors have a point: Why alert people to a disease that they can do nothing about? Unfortunately, this leads people to claim cures when there are none, or at least not everybody can be cured. By writing only about diseases that supposedly can be prevented or cured, magazines give the impression that all diseases can, leading to the widespread mind-set that if you get sick and the doctor cannot diagnose and cure your illness, there's something wrong with the doctor.

While this optimistic bias is undoubtedly partly due to American culture, it is reinforced by advertisers. According to Gloria Steinem, in the days when *Ms.* magazine used to accept ads, it had to convince advertisers that it had an upbeat editorial content. When *Ms.* ran an article on cosmetic surgery showing pictures of some of the bad results, many advertisers—not necessarily cosmetic surgeons—pulled their ads from future issues.

There is more direct pressure from advertisers concerning specific products. When the editor of a magazine for parents of young children suggested that its advertisers were requesting an article on calcium, I countered with a suggestion that several studies had just come out showing that cold remedies really didn't help children feel that much better during colds and that they certainly didn't shorten the cold's duration. This article, I suggested, ought to be of interest to parents, since colds are certainly widespread even if they aren't serious. I had noticed that the manufacturers of some of the cold remedies were advertisers, and the editor called me, good-naturedly, a "troublemaker." Despite the good nature, it was clear to me he didn't want an article that would have alienated advertisers.

The degree of editorial pressure advertisers can bring to bear on a magazine is perhaps most visible—or invisible, as the case may be—among magazines that carry cigarette advertising. In January 1992 researchers from the University of Michigan published in the *New England Journal of Medicine* the results of a detailed survey of 99 U.S. magazines published from 1959 through 1986. "We have found that the higher the percentage of cigarette advertising revenues, the lower the likelihood that a magazine will publish an article on the dangers of smoking," said Prof. Kenneth E. Warner, chairman of public health policy and administration at the University of Michigan and an author of the report. "That is a statistically significant finding." But as the *New York Times* reported, the researchers could not prove definitively that these results were caused by advertising pressures; the researchers were convinced, however, by a "wealth of anecdotal evidence" that such pressures were brought to bear. "Almost all the journalists who will speak to me off the record will acknowledge that this phenomenon exists," Prof. Warner said. "If they speak on the record, they will deny it."

Advertisers aren't the only influence. Many free-lance, and some salaried, journalists accept work from pharmaceutical companies or other interest groups at the same time they are writing for magazines and newspapers. As a catalog for the Learning Annex advertised its three-hour course on "Break into Health and Medical Writing" in the fall of 1991: "Where the big money is (two words—drug companies)." I don't want to be too critical of this practice, because I realize how hard it is to make a living free-lancing. But most free-lance journalists "recycle" material to try to get paid more than once for the same research. If you've just done a pamphlet for a drug company about its new drug for sleep disorders, there will be a tendency to want to earn a bit more by rewriting the information for a consumer magazine. Since most of the sources and information you already have support the company line, the consumer article will probably have that slant, too.

An even more questionable practice is to be paid by a company to place an article as if you were an independent journalist, thereby getting paid twice for it. Such articles should bear the warning that they have been paid for by such-and-such, but they probably never will, since no magazine would be caught dead knowingly telling its readers that they were getting the company line, directly.

Many TV stations, however, are running medical features that come directly from drug companies. While the FDA is now demanding to review such features to make certain they don't advertise unapproved uses of drugs, the fact that stations allow such practices at all could crowd out legitimate medical news that has a chance of being unbiased—features for which the station has to pay—and allow thinly disguised pro-drug ads, which are provided to the stations free of charge, to take over. As Jim Mitchell, an anchor with WDRB-TV News in Louisville, Kentucky, wrote to the *New York Times*: "At many local TV stations, so-called health reporters are merely shills for medical advertisers. As strapped stations grow increasingly desperate for cash flow, some have taken to selling health segments. The advertiser gets not only a conventional commercial but a 'news report' about its product or service. A hospital, pushing its cardiac care unit, will sponsor a 'news story' on heart disease; a psychiatric clinic will bring you a five-part series on teenage depression. . . . Audiences should be aware that the medical 'news' they see may not be news at all, but merely an elaborately faked advertisement."

Drug companies also influence reporting on medical issues by offering prizes to journalists who write about particular subjects. Supposedly the journalists can write about the subject in any way they please. But the William Harvey prize (paid for by Squibb pharmaceuticals, which makes drugs for the treatment of high blood pressure) at one point had as its express purpose the promotion of hypertension as America's number one killer. While the announcement for the prize has since been toned down, it still doesn't encourage stories, for example, including information to show that treatment of mild hypertension has a negligible effect on mortality.

HEALTH EDUCATORS/PROMOTERS

While much of the information people get about health comes from newspapers, much also comes from people who call themselves health educators. Like journalists, this is a group poorly defined by its training: some are physicians, and some are people with little formal training. In theory, the idea of health educators is clearly good, and I'm sure some of the health education they promulgate is sound, too. But in practice there are problems.

- In very few cases is there good proof that following a certain course of action will actually lead to better health. As with medical testing, preventive medicine is largely unregulated, with all sorts of claims being made that are unsupported by the scientific evidence. Dr. Petr Skrabanek, for example, somewhat of a maverick professor of preventive medicine in Ireland, has proposed that health promotion, and particularly experiments in health promotion, should be as subject to ethical scrutiny as any other aspect of health care.

• Because of this, the success of health education must often be judged not by whether people are actually living longer and better, but by how successfully health educators change people's behavior in ways that *might* improve their health, even if there's no good evidence that they actually do. Health educators are judged by how successful they are in getting people to know their cholesterol level or to practice breast self-examination, even though there's not much evidence that such behavior really helps anything in the long run.

• Health education is usually disease-specific, meaning that the health educator must convince patients that the particular disease they are educating about is widespread and serious, since unless they do, there is little justification for their job. Rather than providing people with general information on how to be healthy, which is usually quite simple, health education often takes the form of identifying individuals with risk factors and convincing them of the "seriousness" of their disease. This may lead to a distortion, causing people to worry about things that really aren't that important. A woman whose only risk factor for heart disease, for example, is a slightly elevated blood pressure, probably should just be assured that her risk is not very great and perhaps encouraged to exercise mildly and eat healthily. But health education for high blood pressure has tended to emphasize its seriousness at whatever level, regardless of the absolute risk of serious consequences.

• Some health promotors see their roles as salespeople. Gill Williams of Chelsea College, London University, points out that until there is unequivocal evidence that certain practices will lead to health, "health promotion" is either a meaningless slogan that does not merit serious attention—much less funding—or it is a hard-sell technique that means customers are entitled to consumer protection from sharp practice, exploitation or harm— features noticeably absent at present. As Williams wrote in the *Journal of Medical Ethics*, "Health promotion has none of the safeguards built into it that we have come to expect from other kinds of investments; indeed, health salesmen have so little evidence for their claims and can offer so few guarantees that they would be unlikely to make a living as insurance brokers or the like."

THE PHARMACEUTICAL INDUSTRY

One industry with the strongest interest in convincing people that they're really sick is the pharmaceutical industry, which can sell drugs only if people and their doctors are made to believe they need them. The industry makes its largest profits from drugs that can be sold to large numbers of people and does particularly well with products that can be promoted to healthy people, such as the use of hormone therapy by women in the menopause, since most people are basically well most of the time, even though they can be easily convinced that they are not.

The pharmaceutical industry promotes common problems with multiple causes, such as insomnia and anxiety, as ailments to be cured with drugs. While some people would say that if the treatment's side effects are more severe than the original disease, then the disease should probably not be treated, the pharmaceutical industry tends to see side effects as new marketing opportunities: keep selling the drug, and start promoting another drug to treat the side effects. The drugs commonly prescribed for arthritis, for example, cause gastrointestinal bleeding and sometimes ulcers, and the answer from the pharmaceutical industry has been to promote another drug supposedly to protect the stomach.

Sometimes the fact that people are taking drugs marketed by one company is taken by another as a sign of widespread disease. The Glaxo Institute for Digestive Health, for example, held a press conference in the spring of 1991, citing a statistic from a survey it had commissioned that 17 million Americans took over-the-counter antacids twice a week or more and that these people obviously needed to see a doctor about their heartburn (Glaxo markets a drug prescribed by doctors for stomach problems). What Glaxo hadn't compensated for in the survey was how many of the 17 million might be taking the antacids because *another* drug company was promoting its antacid as a calcium source to be taken by menopausal women to delay the bone-thinning of osteoporosis.

The pharmaceutical industry is the most profitable industry in the United States. Sales by the 100 companies belonging to the Pharmaceutical Manufacturers Association (PMA) topped $32.4 billion in 1989. At least $5 billion of the total sales revenues was spent on marketing, which breaks down to more than $8,000 per allopathic and osteopathic physician in the United States. This enormous amount of money supports activities that have ranged from lavish parties and awarding frequent-flier points to physicians every time they prescribe a particular drug to financing a good number of the newspapers, magazines, and journals received by doctors, as well as sponsoring medical education events. One company offered physicians $100 simply to read the company's literature that encouraged the prescribing of a highly toxic drug for a use that was not approved by the FDA; another company offered $20,000 to a researcher if he could get a seemingly responsible—and positive—study on one of its products published in a major medical journal.

While recent statements by both the American College of Physicians and the American Medical Association have called for a limitation of the more flamboyant marketing procedures, it may be the seemingly innocent "educational" activities that are the most insidious. From 1975 to 1988, the funding of symposia by just 16 companies jumped from $6 million (adjusted for inflation), supporting some 7,519 symposia, to $86 million, supporting some 34,688 symposia, a 14-fold increase in money spent.

Some companies give money with no strings attached. But most pharmaceutical companies tend to support the meetings and investigators that will be favorable to their products and give opportunities for promoting them. Majorie A. Bowman, M.D., director of the Division of Family Practice at Georgetown University School of Medicine, compared mentions of particular drugs during two different drug company-sponsored symposia and found that the company drug was more likely to receive favorable mentions than rival drugs, and "the few statements directly comparing the drugs usually indicated that the company drug was the better drug." While the late Pierre Garai, an advertising executive and a staunch supporter of the pharmaceutical industry, was speaking of advertising when he wrote the following, it probably reflects a mind-set that can be more widely generalized: "The goal of promotion even when travelling under a circuitous path under the guise of 'education' is to achieve uncritical acceptance of a preconceived message—to captivate the mind; stimulation of skeptical thinking would block the purpose."

Drug firms naturally prefer to give a platform to doctors whose views are in line with the company's interests. The FDA's new commissioner, David A. Kessler, M.D., who is cracking down on some of these practices, points out in the *New England Journal of Medicine* that the issue of control can be subtle. "Although most physicians would bridle at having words put into their mouths, they may be tempted to save time by accepting a pharmaceutical company's offer to suggest participants for a symposium, draft a journal article, or prepare slides for a presentation."

The pharmaceutical firms *do* tend to control the subjects of the symposia. James H. Sanders, M.D., a family practitioner in Brevard, North Carolina, a mountain town of about 5,000, says that physicians in his area are always glad to have contact with medical speakers sent in from places such as Duke University. The doctors brought in are good speakers and sincere about what they are saying. But the subjects of such symposia, which often include a dinner, nearly always have something to do with a drug that a particular company is promoting. Dr. Sanders says, "We're getting a lot of education about drug treatment of illness, but we don't get much about public health, we don't get much about radiology, and we sure don't get much about alcohol and drug abuse."

One expert on alcohol and drug abuse, Dr. Sanders reports, was invited to speak, and then was asked by the organization's sponsor what drugs he would talk about so they could find a drug company to sponsor the meeting. When the expert replied that he was trying to get addicted people off prescription drugs, rather than on them, he found his invitation was revoked. Dr. Sanders adds that such "educational" seminars do sometimes underestimate the risks of treatment with the drugs under question. Xanax, for example, was promoted as the drug of first choice in panic disorders and as a drug that could be taken indefinitely. But Xanax is not generally recognized as the first choice for treatment, he pointed out, and it can cause people to become addicted.

Ralph Lach, M.D., director of the Adult Cardiovascular Training Program at Mount Carmel Medical Center in Columbus, Ohio, who has been critical of drug treatment for high cholesterol, points out that dissenters like himself are suppressed in a passive fashion. "When I speak about the lack of evidence of benefit for cholesterol-lowering drugs, my honorarium is nonexistent. Procholesterol people would be supported by the pharmaceutical industry. There's no forum for the anticholesterol viewpoint."

The drug industry spends $350 million a year advertising its products in medical journals. Physicians often deny being in any way influenced by such advertisements, but Jerry Avorn, M.D., and his colleagues at Harvard Medical School found that when a group of doctors were asked about the properties of certain drugs, their answers more closely resembled the information being promulgated in ads than that found in the scientific literature. A recent look at drug advertisements in medical journals showed that indeed there was a significant difference in what a group of expert reviewers thought the ads *should* say and what they actually said. When researchers from UCLA scrutinized 109 ads for prescription drugs that had appeared in 10 leading medical journals, they found that 92 percent violated federal rules created to stop misleading claims. Side effects and contraindications were not highlighted in 47 percent of the ads where the reviewers thought they should have been. In 58 percent of the ads containing images, the reviewers thought that the pictures minimized concerns about side effects. The authors of the study, in selecting their group of reviewers, had initially intended to exclude all experts who had accepted more than $300 from the pharmaceutical industry in the previous two years, but had to drop this requirement because it would have excluded most of the reviewers they had selected. A total of 71 percent of the reviewers had received money from the drug industry, with over half of those receiving more than $5000.

Such ads support a large number of the so-called throwaway publications—newspapers and magazines sent free of charge to members of the medical profession, often based on their prescribing habits. Pathologists, for example, rarely get them because they don't prescribe. I have written for many of these publications myself, and some are quite responsible. But beneath the surface of journalistic objectivity, everyone basically knows that you don't offend the advertisers too much, especially in hard economic times, when advertising revenues are particularly vulnerable. When Arthur M. Sackler was international publisher of *Medical Tribune*, for example, he would periodically assign a writer to do a series attacking the FDA when it took an action that the drug industry—particularly those companies whose drugs were big advertisers in the *Tribune*—perceived as threatening. When I worked for *Rheumatology News*, published independently but under a grant from Syntex pharmaceuticals, I was sometimes asked to cover, supposedly as a journalist, a meeting sponsored by Syntex at which investigators whose work had been sponsored by Syntex would be reporting their results.

The medical journals to which doctors subscribe have a little more independence because their income is more diversified, but they, too, rely heavily on advertising revenues, most of it from pharmaceutical companies. In 1982, for example, the *Journal of the American Medical Association* published a "make-up" news article to appease Pfizer laboratories, which had pulled its advertising to protest an earlier article citing a competitor's drug.

Pharmaceutical companies formerly didn't advertise prescription drugs directly to consumers—not because it was forbidden, but because they were afraid of offending doctors, who, after all, had final control over prescribing the drug, and because the FDA said that all such advertisements must list all the side effects, just as they were required to do when advertising directly to physicians. Pharmaceutical companies were loath to do this, perhaps because all the fine print couldn't be read on television; perhaps because it could.

But in recent years the informal prohibition against advertising to the public has been breaking down. Drug companies spent $70 million advertising prescription drugs to consumers in 1990, up from $40 million in 1989, and industry experts expect the growth to continue. Sometimes the ads present added inducements to take the drug: A 1991 ad in *Parade* offered a number of free and discounted goods and services that people taking the drug

Tenormin, a beta-blocker used in heart patients, could get, including Polaroid film and compact disks.

To get away from the need to list all the side effects, such publicity often takes the form of advertising the *disease* for which the drug is to be prescribed. This tactic has been favored mostly by those companies that market the only product for the disease in question, like Upjohn, which manufactures minoxidil, a drug used in the treatment for baldness. As in most cases of disease mongering, side effects are conveniently left out, as is the fact that minoxidil is effective only in a small percent of men.

The drug industry also supports an extensive network of public relations firms that specialize in medical issues. Sometimes they provide supposedly impartial "backgrounders" about particular diseases, the bias of which becomes apparent upon closer scrutiny. One backgrounder about upper respiratory infections, for example, mentioned that doctors prescribe different antibiotics for different respiratory infections. It left out the fact that many, if not most, upper respiratory infections are caused by viruses, for which antibiotic treatment is useless.

All of these ploys have been very effective. Dr. Ralph Lach considers that "the cholesterol hysteria currently sweeping our country and its physicians is clearly the machination of the pharmaceutical industry." While a health-anxious public, well-intentioned but uninformed do-gooders, and more or less willing physicians have also fueled it, he admits, the greatest zeal "is that of the drug industry, which, according to some, stands to develop a $10-$20 billion-a-year business from its cholesterol scam."

The drug industry has also helped to put a pharmacologic "spin" on many diseases that might be better treated in other ways. Jerry Avorn, M.D., of Harvard Medical School, and his colleagues presented a case report of a patient with abdominal pain to physicians and nurses throughout the country, encouraging them to ask for more information about the patient (the medical history) and give their recommendations for therapy. One-third of the physicians chose to initiate therapy without seeking the relevant history, which included severe psychosocial stress and substantial use of aspirin, coffee, cigarettes, and alcohol. Nearly half of all physicians indicated that a prescription would be the single most effective therapy, with 65 percent recommending an ulcer medication "despite the unproved efficacy of such medications when used to treat abdominal pain without ulcer, as in the case presented." Apparently, wrote Dr. Avorn and his coworkers in *Archives of Internal Medicine*, "quite early in the formulation of the problem, the conceptual focus appears to shift from broader questions like 'What is wrong with this patient?' or 'What can I do to help?' to the much narrower concern, 'Which prescription shall I write?'"

By contrast, only 19 percent of nurse practitioners opted to treat without taking further history, and only 20 percent of the nurses recommended a prescription medication.

But while it is constantly trying to push the limits of its regulation, the drug industry is, at least, regulated. The diagnostics industry, however, is often not.

THE DIAGNOSTICS INDUSTRY

An ad in my neighborhood newspaper says, "Cancer? Infectious disease? Any growing lump anywhere in your body (breast, skin, etc.), rash or temperature elevation may be a cancer or a serious illness that requires immediate expert medical attention." The ad further promises, "If you have insurance coverage and a medical problem, you may be eligible for a complete cancer examination, which will identify almost any serious illness."

"Leg Pain," screeches the inch-high headline, with the rest of the copy then suggesting that such a symptom could be fatal. The advertisement, for a diagnostics center, is using the common disease-mongering tactic, described in chapter 5, of taking a commonly occurring symptom and exaggerating its seriousness. "Without adequate education, and affected by anxiety about possibly serious health problems," wrote Richard J. Feinstein, M.D., in the *Journal of the Florida Medical Association*, "elderly people easily fall prey to those entrepreneurs who own these diagnostic facilities. These facilities exist in a vacuum, outside the traditional locations at hospitals and medical centers." They are particularly common in Florida.

We have already seen that both diagnosis and diagnostic tests require a good deal of intelligence and wisdom, and if they are to be made in the patient's interest, the doctor (and perhaps the patient) must constantly be asking himself or herself whether the benefits to the patient will be worth the risks. But most such centers are not set up to benefit patients: They are set up to make money. It's possible that the rare patient may in fact benefit by having some previously undiagnosed and treatable disease found. But many others will undergo a series of expensive and possibly dangerous tests that may then lead to treatment that does them no good. A center set up to make money diagnosing and treating high blood pressure, for example, is not likely to pay that much attention to caveats about treating blood pressure that is only mildly raised, and in people who have no other risk factors for heart disease.

While a savvy patient can avoid going to freestanding diagnostic centers, it's been harder, at least until recently, to avoid those doctors who operate outside the centers but own a significant proportion of their stock and refer a significant proportion of the patients. Such centers sought out doctors as investors not for their investment capital, which could have been provided by anyone with a little money, but because they were a source of patient referrals. Indeed, they did refer: According to Robert D. Carl III, writing in the *New York Times*, physician-investors speak in terms of "owning patients" and ask "why can't I make a little more money on my patients?" A 1989 study by the Department of Health and Human Services found that patients of referring doctors who invested in clinical labs received 45 percent more services than Medicare patients in general. One estimate was that the cost of spurious magnetic resonance imaging tests alone was $1 billion in 1990.

Health Images Inc., a publicly traded diagnostic imaging center, testified before a congressional subcommittee that when the company had formed joint ventures with doctors in its early years, the physician partners "impeded, rather than facilitated" high-quality care. "Physicians actually objected to the company's spending money for routine upgrades. They argued that such improvements were unnecessary and that the funds could be better used to increase the returns on their investment." After buying out physician joint ventures and examining the medical files, Health Images found significant evidence "that many patients were being referred for unnecessary procedures."

By early 1991, this practice had gotten entirely out of hand:

more than 10 percent of the nation's doctors had invested in businesses to which they referred patients. In Florida, the proportion of doctors making such investments reached 40 percent, with 60 percent of Florida's clinical labs owned by physicians. In the summer of 1991, the regulators clamped down, requiring that doctors who referred patients could own only 40 percent of such joint-ventures, causing them precipitously to rearrange their affairs. In September 1991, the American Medical Association suggested that doctors tell patients if they own part of the diagnostics facilities to which they are referring, although just how the AMA might enforce this suggestion remains to be seen. But while the issue of joint-ventures has received a lot of attention recently, an article in the Hastings Center Report points out that the ethical questions raised by a physician holding stock in a laboratory to which he or she refers patients are really no different than those raised by the physician who perform X rays or other tests in their own offices, and indeed may be less acute. Physicians who own part of the facilities to which they refer patients are getting a margin of profit, but at least they may be referring patients to specialists skilled in interpreting the tests they perform. General physicians who perform X rays in their offices receive all the profits, and are performing tests they probably do not have the training to properly interpret.

Some laboratories are now encouraging the idea that patients should be able to order their own tests. "Many states," wrote Henry B. Soloway, from Associated Pathologists Laboratories in Las Vegas, "already permit consumers to order tests directly on themselves simply by presenting themselves to a laboratory facility of their choice. And this trend is growing." Dr. Soloway, writing in the *Journal of the American Medical Association*, makes the point that from one billion to 1.25 billion lab tests per year are performed in nontraditional settings, with a total price tag as high as $8 billion, and that many of these tests are substandard. "So great is the demand for nontraditional health testing and related medical services that 38 million Americans are estimated to have used some fraudulent health product during the past year, spending $27 billion in the process," according to Dr. Soloway.

"My opinion is that if a consumer with disposable income wishes to spend it on cosmetic surgery, a luxury car, a chemistry

panel, or a Caribbean vacation, he or she should be free to do so,"
wrote Dr. Soloway in answer to the letters responding to his
initial article. The problem is that consumers have at least a
somewhat realistic idea of what a Caribbean vacation, a luxury
car, and perhaps even cosmetic surgery might mean to their lives.
But with testing seen to be much more meaningful than it really
is, people are likely to spend money for what they perceive is
insurance of good health when in fact a battery of tests provides
no guarantees, and can prove harmful.

DOCTORS

Most disease mongering by doctors probably stems from sheer
demographics. The number of doctors (M.D.s and D.O.s) increased 44 percent between 1980 and 1990, while the U.S. population grew by only 10 percent over the same period. On the
average, physicians are seeing 8 percent fewer patients a week
than they were 10 years ago. Physicians in nearly all specialties
were operating at what they judged to be "below capacity,"
including 59 percent of plastic surgeons, 57 percent of general
surgeons, and 33 percent of pediatricians. Thoracic and cardiovascular surgeons said they could handle 30 percent more office
visits. Medicare recently cut its total budget by 6.5 percent, but
said that total payments to doctors would remain unchanged
because, to offset the cut, physicians would increase the number
of patients they see.

Many doctors protest that they are not in the profession just
to make money, although nearly all concede they would like to
be well paid for what they do. But when Arnold S. Relman, M.D.,
former editor of the *New England Journal of Medicine,* wrote, "I
do not believe it [economic reward] is the most important one for
the vast majority of people who go into medicine," Alexander A.
Stemer, M.D., of Munster, Indiana, surveyed ten physicians of his
subspecialty group and found that they were unanimous in their
disagreement. "Although all our physicians value the other re-
wards of practice—most important, fulfillment in doing 'so much
good and [earning] the everlasting gratitude of those being served'—
all indicated that they would not have entered the field of medicine
had they not thought that economic stability was ensured." Alan

P. Zelicoff, M.D., of Albuquerque, New Mexico, pointed out that there are many other careers that lead to immense social usefulness, but they generally pay less. "Like it or not, people—physicians included—are motivated by economic reward." In a letter to the *New England Journal of Medicine*, David M. Battista, M.D., of New York, pointed out that his student loan indebtedness of over $140,000 for his medical education made it difficult for him to be altruistic.

As a result, turf wars—who does what to which patients—have been raging. "With medical supply exceeding demand, with nonmedical healers wanting to graze in the rich fields of third-party payment, jurisdictional disputes are increasing," wrote Walter W. Benjamin in the *New England Journal of Medicine.* "The boundary lines prescribing who can do what are often fuzzy, so that a gynecologic procedure, for example, may be performed by a family practitioner, an obstetrician, a urologist, a general surgeon, or any of a number of other specialists."

Cardiologists, for example, are battling with interventional radiologists and cardiac surgeons to decide who has the right to treat disease of the coronary arteries; as a result the number of angioplasties, which can be performed by any of the three, has risen precipitously. Cardiologists may soon be entering the field of treating narrowings of blood vessels in the arms and legs, a field traditionally divided between vascular surgeons and interventional radiologists. "With the changes in the reimbursement systems," says Ernest Ring, M.D., chief of interventional radiology at the University of California at San Francisco, "everybody will be scurrying around to find things they can do. Peripheral vascular disease symptoms range from the trivial to the severe, and people may begin looking at the anatomy and fixing it whether or not it's important to the patient."

The way we pay doctors in the United States is based on the procedures they perform, and while surgeons make money based on the operations they do, the easiest way for the nonsurgeon to make much money is to perform diagnostic tests. Medical specialists who don't normally perform significant numbers of tests are among the lowest paid. A 1991 study found that even the changes in payment schedule designed to reward doctors' "thinking" relatively more than their doing would not make it worthwhile to invest in training in rheumatology, a specialty in which relatively few procedures are performed. The specialty of gastroenterology, however, with its numerous tests, more than paid for the cost of the training. Noninvasive doctors can invest in office testing equipment, which means they can charge for the tests they do, and the volume of testing in doctors' offices is increasing by 15 percent annually. No wonder sales of medical testing equipment and supplies for the doctor's office, which exceeded $1.2 billion in 1987 are projected to more than double in the next five years. Besides producing income for the diagnosing physician, "surgeons and other specialists win because the tests find extra patients for them," said Frank von Richter, vice president of Boston Biomedical.

A brochure from Life Sciences, Inc., for example, tells doctors how much they can expect to make on their patients if they lease a number of devices designed to check the status of the patient's vascular system. The system costs $1,883.50 per month to lease, but even if the doctor does only ten tests a week, according to the brochure, he or she increases the net profit to the yearly practice, after one year, by $12,100. If the doctor performs 50 tests a week, he or she earns $412,100 extra each year. The brochure provides sample diagnostic codes that can be used to justify the procedures—for example, varicose veins of the lower extremity without ulcer and without inflammation.

THE LAWYERS AND THE COURTS

Doctors rationalize their large amount of testing as "defensive medicine" and admit that while the chances that the testing will benefit their patients are small, if they are ever sued for malpractice, they will be able to show that they did everything they could.

There is a certain amount of truth in this. Elsa Shartsis, a lawyer from the Detroit area (who is married to a physician) says that when she used to work on malpractice cases, the first thing she did was to subpoena the records and look for things that should have been done and weren't. In response to an article in the *Journal of American Medical Association* showing that electronic fetal monitoring increased the rate of cesarean sections but didn't decrease the rate of babies who died or had birth defects, Morris Wizenberg, M.D., wrote: "Electronic fetal monitoring may well be expensive and useless, but regardless of what the recommendations of physicians may be, until the courts accept a similar position, obstetricians abandon the procedure only at their own peril."

While one can be somewhat sympathetic with physicians on this point, their problem may be that they are listening too closely to the lawyers they despise. Lawyers have an interest in telling doctors how to defend themselves if faced with a malpractice suit, which probably means documenting that everything possible was done. But most lawyers don't have an interest in telling doctors how to *prevent* a lawsuit from being brought in the first place, because then the lawyers themselves would suffer financially.

Preventing the suits from being brought in the first place is probably more important than being prepared to defend yourself, since by and large patients who sue have not necessarily been injured, but are for some reason angry at the doctor. Several recent studies have shown that very few patients who have been injured as a result of medical care actually sue; one study found one in ten injured patients did so, and another found that only 1.5 percent of patients who had been injured in a hospital brought suit. Some patients who aren't really injured sue anyway, and here again the "niceness" factor probably plays a big role. In addition, few doctors actually lose when a case is brought against them. Many observers, therefore, believe that doctors can best defend themselves from lawsuits not by mindlessly performing tests and procedures on their patients, but by learning to talk to them, being attentive and sympathetic, and giving full explanations of what the patients' choices are and what the consequences will be. "The best legal protection for the obstetricians is informed consent," wrote Stephen B. Thacker and H. David Banta in response to Dr. Wizenberg's letter.

Gunnar B. Stickler, M.D., retired former chairman and professor of pediatrics at the Mayo Clinic in Rochester, Minnesota, says, "If you practice to protect yourself, that is malpractice." Dr. Stickler says he always tried to arrange for a minimum number of tests and to use only proven therapies. He was never sued for malpractice in his 40 years of practicing medicine in the United States, although the father of a teenage girl did report him to the state medical board for diagnosing her as having a psychosomatic illness. The threat of a malpractice suit, then, while real, is exaggerated, and physicians often use it as an excuse to perform tests that benefit them financially. Uwe E. Reinhardt, James Madison Professor of Political Economy at Princeton University, says that "the greatest boon to a physician's income is the malpractice excuse. I don't think that if malpractice were reformed it would make even a dent in health costs."

HOSPITALS

During the past decade, the federal government, through Medicare, decided to change the way hospitals were paid. Instead of paying hospitals for the number of days a patient was hospitalized and for each procedure performed, the government decided to institute a system of prospective payment known as diagnosis-related groups (DRGs), where the hospital would be paid a set sum based on the patient's diagnosis, and no more. I've already discussed some of the intellectual problems of making diagnosis the basis of the payment system and the fact that they are constantly being adjusted for seriousness. From a practical point of view, DRGs have meant that hospitals had to change the way they balanced their budgets. Rather than performing more procedures on the same patient or keeping the patient in the hospital for more days, the hospital now had two different incentives: to attempt to assign the DRG (read "diagnosis") that was reimbursed at the highest rate, and to bring in new patients, preferably ones with a high DRG reimbursement level who didn't need high levels of care. While one satirist suggested that the best way to do the latter was to start admitting dead patients, who after all would need by way of care only occasional swabbing down with disinfectant, the other possibility was to admit healthy patients and give them the worst possible diagnosis that could be defended. At least one New York hospital offers ambulance drivers bonuses if they bring insured patients to that hospital.

Soon after the institution of DRGs, computer programs were developed to help find the most severe diagnosis in order to get maximum reimbursement, a phenomenon dubbed "DRG creep." Donald W. Simborg, M.D., who coined the term in 1981, wrote in the *New England Journal of Medicine*, "When does abdominal pain and duodenal scarring on an upper-gastrointestinal-tract series become the more costly 'probable duodenal ulcer'? When does 'probable transient ischemic attack' become the much more costly 'possible stroke'?" Simborg also predicted that DRGs would reinforce the tendency to do more and more diagnostic tests: "There will be incentives to look a little harder and to perform that extra test or procedures to make a diagnosis."

Dr. Simborg's prediction proved true. Dorothy Thompson, M.B., an English doctor working in Texas, wrote that "attempts are often made to add to, or subtly change the doctor's final diagnosis so that they can charge insurance companies more—for example, adding a diagnosis of jaundice to hyperbilirubinemia." Susan Horn, Ph.D., of the Johns Hopkins School of Public Health found that DRGs were in many cases doing more than creeping: they were leaping. While reviewing hospital records, she found that many patients coded as having either shock or heart attacks—both of which pay well under DRGs—had symptoms consistent with neither. It was for this reason, she explained, that a National Institutes of Health (NIH) conference found dramatic differences in the survival rates for shock, which varied from 30 to 90 percent from hospital to hospital. "Where they had 90 percent survival," says Dr. Horn, "the patients really weren't in shock." Lisa I. Iezzoni, M.D., and her coworkers of Boston University Medical Center, found that teaching hospitals in particular were likely to assign the code for myocardial infarction (heart attack) to patients who either didn't have or weren't receiving treatment for this condition: 41.7 percent of patients in "tertiary," or referral teaching, hospitals, had been assigned a code indicating acute myocardial infarction when in fact they weren't being treated for that, compared with 9.1 percent at nonteaching facilities.

If a hospital realizes that it is having trouble meeting its budget, it may decide it needs to perform more cardiac surgery, a major breadwinner for hospitals. "There is some conventional wisdom in healthcare that says as cardiology goes, so goes the rest of the hospital business," wrote one healthcare marketing consultant.

For example, the Health Care Advisory Board in Washington calculated a few years ago that a single cardiac surgery has a net marginal profit per patient of $4,049. But in order to get patients eligible for cardiac surgery, hospitals first have to provide the diagnostic tests that will funnel the patients into surgery, in this case cardiac catheterization. One hospital in Montana found it must complete ten catheterizations to "achieve" one surgery. A hospital in Alabama, which had a decline in net revenue from total cardiac services, was able to increase its catheterizations by 10 percent in six months through the use of simple screening tests administered by referring physicians in conjunction with their heart specialists. "Begin by calculating your ratios of catheterizations to surgeries and then establish positive means for filling the top of the funnel through higher use of diagnostic procedures," wrote the consultant. One hospital did this by placing a board-certified cardiologist from the medical center to act on a part-time basis as a consultant for the local internists. Other hospitals establish "feeders" of ambulatory satellites, dispersed clinics, and preferred provider organizations (where patients are funneled to the hospital's doctors) and even go after patients with helicopters.

All this would be well and good if disease were a finite thing and all you had to do was go out and search for what was currently not being treated. But remember that the indications for catheterization are not cut-and-dried, nor are the indications for surgery, with the Rand Corporation finding that 37 to 78 percent of the cases ranked as inappropriate when viewed from hospital to hospital. A system that works by calculating first how many heart surgeries it must perform to balance its budget (or make a profit), then going out in search of bodies upon which to perform them, is hardly likely to use very strict criteria in deciding who will benefit from catherization or from the subsequent surgery. No matter that women tend to have a high rate of false positives on stress testing: a hospital trying to perform more catheterizations is hardly likely to mind. No matter that many chest pains are a reflection of anxiety or illness having nothing to do with the heart, or that most cardiac bypasses are performed to improve the quality of life, not to lengthen it, and a judgment of improving its quality can be made only after a careful discussion with the patient. Such considerations are important only to the patient, who conveniently gets left out of the cost-benefit ratio.

DRGs are not the only problem. E. Haavi Morreim, of the

University of Tennessee School of Medicine at Memphis, points out that in psychiatry, DRGs have not yet been imposed. Here, the number of hospital beds has generally expanded: between 1970 and 1986, the proportion of proprietary inpatient psychiatric beds multiplied by a factor of 15; the number of freestanding psychiatric hospitals has grown dramatically, as has the number of psychiatric units in general community hospitals. At the same time, insurance coverage for mental health has been expanding. "As the number of inpatient beds rises to greet their new-found insurance coverage," Morreim wrote in the *Journal of Medicine and Philosophy*, "commensurate pressures arise to find lots of mentally ill people to fill them. Psychiatry therefore is encouraged to expand the number and scope of mental illness diagnoses."

NATIONAL ORGANIZATIONS

National organizations such as the National Institutes of Health, the American Cancer Society, and the American Heart Association have a tough job: Americans don't like to admit that some diseases can't be cured with present medical techniques and knowledge. This attitude may pay off in the long term; perhaps a can-do attitude will eventually defeat all obstacles to come up with a cure. But in the short term, it puts the heads of these organizations on the horns of a dilemma. What happens when a major study shows that a treatment they are advocating doesn't work? For organizations such as the National Institutes of Health (NIH), which draw heavily on taxpayers' money, they cannot really go to Congress and say, "This approach didn't work and we're back to square zero"—at least if they want to keep their jobs. What happens, then, is that such leaders interpret the studies in ways that show that they worked, at least in some patients, or that the treatments would work if only people could be made to behave.

When several major studies, for example, showed that treatment to lower cholesterol might prevent a few deaths from heart attack but increased deaths from other causes so that the total death rate was not lowered at all, the response of the National

Heart, Lung, and Blood Institute was not to go slow on cholesterol but instead to launch a massive campaign to get all Americans to know their blood cholesterol level. When the special advisory panel of doctors failed to endorse this approach, since the evidence that it would do any good was so slight, some of the panel members claimed that their grant applications were no longer approved by NIH.

Similarly the American Cancer Society recommends mammography screening of women between the ages of 40 and 50, even though most studies have shown that such screening does not reduce the death rate from breast cancer in women in this age group. Preliminary reports from Canada indicate that adding mammography to breast examination may actually increase deaths from breast cancer in women between the ages of 40 and 50. But the society's advisers who took a more cautious approach to screening this age group found they were not invited back.

According to a former director of the U.S. White House Drug Policy Office, Carlton Turner, Ph.D., illicit drug use in the United States has consistently declined for the past decade, but nobody wants to admit it.

"By every measurable and objective role we know drug use is down overall, but nobody wants to admit it because everyone's budget is driven by the drug problem," Dr. Turner told *The Journal of the Addiction Research Foundation of Ontario*. "You have no organized group with a vested interest in seeing drug abuse go away, except, perhaps, the parents."

PATIENTS

I have always been a fan of the idea of patient groups, since patients can exchange information about their disease and information about doctors and generally cry on each other's shoulders. While researching a book on hysterectomy, I attended some sessions of the Endometriosis Association of Greater New York and was so impressed that I was *almost* sorry I didn't have endometriosis myself.

But some patients and patient advocates like to proselytize their disease for certain psychological gratification. They, too, have an interest in making you think you are sick. One reason is commendable: they themselves were misunderstood before they got their diagnosis, which was a great relief. They would like you to benefit from the same relief. They therefore promulgate the symptoms of their "disease" so that others can benefit from finding out what is causing their symptoms, as they did. Unfortunately, very few symptoms are highly specific for a given disease, and most of these efforts end up suggesting that non-specific symptoms such as fatigue mean you have the disease in question.

Some of the patient groups receive financial support from people who make drugs to treat the disease. Barry Werth reported in the *New York Times Magazine* that the Human Growth Foundation, a nonprofit advocacy group for short children, receives two-thirds of its national budget from Genentech and Eli Lilly, both of which market hormones to treat short children.

Another reason patients and patient advocates want you to feel that you, too, could get the disease is to try to remove the stigma of certain diseases such as AIDS. Thus messages such as "All women can get AIDS" are promoted to try to get people to think it's not just IV drug users who can be "blamed" for getting their disease and therefore marginalized. While the message is technically accurate—all women *can* get AIDS, if they are exposed to the virus either sexually or intravenously—it fails to put into perspective the point that many women are extremely unlikely to. Most women with AIDS at the time of this writing were either IV drug users or partners of IV drug users, and the monogamous spouse of a monogamous husband who did not use IV drugs still remained at a risk of infection that was practically nil. The strategy of telling all people that they, too, could get AIDS may have backfired in its plan to stop stigmatizing AIDS victims. Telling people that they, too, can get AIDS may simply make them more threatened, more irrational, and more willing to support repressive laws to try to stem the spread of the virus.

In the addictions area, people who consider themselves "addicted" to food or sex or "addicted" as codependents may be particularly vocal in trying to convince you that you, too, have a disease. Everyone has to eat, and some people enjoy food, causing them to give it a large importance in their life. Those so inclined might consider them "addicted to food." "People who have messed their lives up most corner the market in expressing their points of view. . . . You might say we are spreading the most unhealthy point of view," says Stanton Peele. "Problem people have cornered the market."

WORKER'S COMPENSATION

Nortin Hadler, M.D., a professor of rheumatology at the University of North Carolina, points out that the process of getting compensation for a work-related illness or injury is a process of learning to be a patient. Getting pain in one's hands or shoulders, for example, quite commonly follows from having to perform tasks repetitively, and the best cure is to find a way to rest the joints that are being overworked. If your workplace does not allow for this—does not allow, for example, adequate work breaks or ways to change the stresses—and you apply for worker's compensation, you then have to put a name to your "disease," the most common of which is repetitive strain injury or thoracic outlet syndrome. If the pain is in your back, rather than being allowed the time that will let it go away and allow you to continue working, you may have to prove that you "injured" your back, whereas in reality most backaches, like most headaches, don't result at all from injuries. Once you get a diagnosis such as carpal tunnel syndrome or repetitive strain injury, you may become a candidate for surgery, which may cause its own complications and won't help at all if you have to go back to the same work environment. You have thus been converted from a patient with a slight and curable ailment to one with an incurable disease.

HEALTH AND LIFE INSURANCE COMPANIES

Health insurers may be the only player with an interest in not making you sick—once you have been accepted for insurance. But until you have been judged healthy enough to be accepted for insurance in this strange system of ours in which only the healthy can get health insurance, they are absolutely brilliant at converting what would otherwise be trivial illnesses into life-threatening ones. While working on this book, I received a call from someone trying to get me to switch my policy from Blue Cross. But when she found out I had fibroid tumors—a very common and benign condition of many women—she immediately advised me to stay with Blue Cross. My benign condition was suddenly made to sound serious, and if I hadn't already done a lot of research about fibroids, I might have been inclined to accept her assessment that I had a seemingly serious disease—at least from the standpoint of insurance.

Risk rating, in fact, is a major reason that more and more middle-class people are without health insurance.

Seven million Americans have been refused medical insurance because of a medical condition, trivial or not. And this number grossly understates the number of Americans who are affected by risk-rating, since many are staying with jobs they dislike because they know they would have difficulty getting individual coverage. A 1991 *New York Times*-CBS poll of Americans showed that three of ten said they or others in their household remained with jobs they wished to leave because of health insurance benefits, a phenomenon that has come to known as "job lock."

There's another, more subtle way that insurance companies tend to add to the numbers of well people who think they are sick. Joyce R. Adamson, M.D., of Stoneham, Massachusetts, points out in a letter to *Archives of Internal Medicine* that "some insurance companies will not pay for more than three separate tests, because it is cheaper to order a whole chemistry profile." What inevitably happens, she says, is that if the doctor wants to follow four different levels, say in a patient with hypertension, the doctor must order an entire profile. This leads to other abnormalities turning up that are probably unimportant but have to be followed up, nevertheless.

OTHERS

Other, relatively minor players may factor in a given disease. The food industry has played a major role in the diseasing of high cholesterol, and manufacturers of tick repellant have been responsible for some of the frightening images of Lyme disease.

Disease mongering attracts even the small-time entrepreneur: anybody in New York City who owns a sphygmomanometer may set up on a busy street corner to convince you, in exchange for a small donation or perhaps a conversion to vegetarianism, that you have high blood pressure. To name all the players would be exhausting and counterproductive. What is more important is to study their tactics and to learn how to decode their messages so you can decide if what is obviously going to benefit them will also benefit you.

Chapter 5

Disease-Mongering Tactics

Manipulation of competition may be considered the last refuge of the scoundrel in medicine and surgery.
—Melvin A. Block, M.D., *Archives of Surgery*, 1989.

We may very well have nothing to fear but fear itself, but we do have fear itself.
—Henry Allen, *Newsday*, 1990.

It was not that unusual as meetings go: several doctors and researchers had convened to talk about premenstrual syndrome (PMS), and according to the invitation, the sponsor was an eminent southern university. During the question-and-answer sessions, however, a doctor asked the following "question": 20 to 40 percent of women "suffered" from the bloating of PMS, he said, and the American College of Obstetricians and Gynecologists had recommended that such women should be treated with spironolactone, a diuretic. Any experienced medical journalist by now recognized that this man was obviously a plant; while the meeting was nominally sponsored by a university, it was really sponsored by a drug company that manufactured spironolactone. In case we didn't get the point, the lunchtime speaker, a former Olympic gymnast, gave an added plug for the drug.

A few days later, while flipping through some medical journals, I discovered that spironolactone is a suspected carcinogen. In England, it is not authorized for the treatment of high blood pressure for this reason. Even the *U.S. Physicians Desk Reference*, which contains information provided by the manufacturer, says, in bold type, "Warning: Spironolactone, an ingredient of Aldactazide, has been shown to be a tumorigen in chronic toxicity studies in rats (see Warnings). Aldactazide should be used only in those conditions described under Indications and Usage. Unnecessary use of this drug should be avoided."

If we define disease mongering as exaggerating the severity of the disease and minimizing the side effects of treatment, this has to be a classic example. Let's analyze this incident more closely, for in these few minutes of questioning, the plant used many of the techniques classically used by disease-mongers.

• *Taking a normal function and implying that there's something wrong with it and it should be treated.* In social science jargon this is known as "medicalization." Now it's true that many women bloat in the week before their menstruation begins: that's normal physiology. By pointing it out in the way he did, the plant was implying that there was something wrong with premenstrual bloating. Medicalization is an often-used disease-mongering tactic; other conditions often "medicalized" are menopause, shortness in children, "malocclusion," childbirth, and obesity. Implying that something essentially normal is a disease is a prime tactic. About 90 percent of women will have irregular menstrual periods as they approach menopause, yet one Chicago woman reports her doctor told her (in trying to convince her to have a hysterectomy for her abnormal bleeding) that "a normal menopause in a woman is that your periods stop. That's it."

Another aspect of medicalization is taking problems of everyday life and implying that the doctor has a solution. A news release from Upjohn on stress, for example, lists the signs of stress, including some physical ones but also "emotional and social isolation," "not taking time for oneself in terms of leisure, proper diet, rest, and exercise," "job frustration," and "chronically hostile or angry feelings." "Persistence of any of these symptoms calls for a visit to the doctor," the release tells us, failing to explain that most doctors have not been trained to deal with things like job frustration or not taking enough time for oneself and that some will undoubtedly prescribe a tranquilizer—perhaps one made by Upjohn.

• *Imputing suffering that isn't necessarily there.* It's true that if people are really suffering from normal functions, they may well want treatment. Menstrual cramps, for example, are usually one sign that a woman is ovulating normally, but if they are severe, many women want painkillers instead of a lecture about physiology. But to say someone "suffers" from something is different from saying that someone "experiences" it, and while some of that 20 to 40 percent mentioned by the drug company's plant may really suffer, many others may just notice that they bloat a bit. Be suspicious of disease-mongers who purportedly sympathize so much with others; bloating might just as well be relieved by getting larger clothes as by medications that are suspected carcinogens, and I suspect most women, given adequate information, would choose the clothes.

The tactic of imputing suffering seems to be particularly used by male doctors when trying to justify their treatment of female patients with operations such as hysterectomy or cesarean section. "Why should the modern woman undergo the sweaty, gut-wrenching ordeal of labor that may last 12 to 24 hours or more?" wrote a general surgeon (who did not perform cesarean sections) in the *Journal of the American Medical Association*. "I think the goal should be for all women to give birth by cesarean section." When you talk to women about their hysterectomies or cesareans, the picture becomes more complex: some may have found that the operation relieved their suffering while others found that it caused them to suffer more.

• *Defining as large a proportion of the population as possible as suffering from the "disease."* It was evident from the speeches given at the meeting that although 20 to 40 percent of women may bloat, a much smaller percentage, something under 5 percent, have trouble functioning prior to their periods. The problem is not bloating; it's the mood changes. While spironolactone may help with bloating, it does nothing to relieve negative mood.

The advantages of this tactic to a drug company are evident—a drug that can be marketed for a large proportion of the population is going to produce bigger profits than a drug that is pushed only for those patients who might truly benefit from it.

Pharmaceutical companies seem to love this tactic particularly because it is more "gentlemanly" than attacking the drugs of a competitor. Defining the pie as large as possible, rather than fighting for your share of it, can be masked as a noble attempt to educate the public about their health rather than cut-throat competition.

This tactic can be observed particularly in "threshold diseases" such as high blood pressure and high cholesterol where the line between normal and "diseased" is arbitrary. Just defining the level at which blood pressure becomes "high" at a diastolic of 90 rather than 95, for example, doubles the population labeled as having high blood pressure, since relatively few people have levels above 95 and a great many have levels between 90 and 95.

Not only drug companies have an interest in making the problem seem as widespread as possible. If you're head of one of the National Institutes of Health, for example, you hardly have an interest in defining a disease in a narrow way that means only a few people have it: How can you justify your budget that way?

Journalists are also particularly susceptible to this tactic, since it is much easier to sell an editor on a disease that affects 25 percent of the population than on a drug that affects only 1 percent. One woman I know is trying to sell a book that says mitral valve prolapse is a serious disease that affects 20 percent of women, a case of trying to eat your cake and have it too. If you define a disease like mitral valve prolapse in a way that includes a large percentage of the population, you're defining it in a way where the condition in many people will be trivial. If you define it in a narrow way, taking only those people in whom it is a fairly serious condition, only a small percentage of the population will be affected. You can't realistically have it both ways. Yet mongers will try, using the most serious definition of the disease applied to the largest number of people.

This can create an unholy alliance, with pharmaceutical companies, specialist groups, and others putting out figures of how common a disease is and the press having an incentive *not* to check them out too carefully for fear that their story will evaporate. As Dr. Jean-Charles Sournia wrote a few years ago, speaking of the situation in France, "Most of the impressive [mortality] statistics provided to the press by heart specialists about heart disease, by lung specialists about lung disease, or specialists of ski, judo, or 'jerk' accidents are without scientific justification, most of the time enlarged in good faith: everyone preaches for his saint. If you added up all the mortalities supplied by each medical specialty, you'd get double the true mortality!" A 1991 press release from Wang Associates, for example, a public relations firm, notes that 50 million Americans suffer from at least one bout of insomnia each year and that a new medication for short-term insomnia, ProSom, has just been approved by the FDA. Now for most of us, one bout of insomnia a year is not exactly something to become worried about; many of us do our most creative thinking while lying awake in bed. As "Minerva" in the *British Medical Journal* noted about another press release on insomnia, "An Upjohn leaflet for the press informs us that Napoleon, Dickens, Churchill, Kafka, Kipling, Proust, Edison, and Van Gogh were all insomniacs. Perhaps instead of treating insomnia doctors should be encouraging it."

• *Conveniently forgetting to mention side effects.* In the case of the PMS meeting, this was a particularly egregious omission. Even if the carcinogenicity was only suspected, it's a pretty serious side effect for a drug that treats a normal condition that doesn't even bother most people that much. Yet I know of no one who has been given any idea of what side effects might occur when they undergo surgery, and people don't usually know them when doctors prescribe a drug. While drug advertisements for prescription drugs must give side effects (in small print), those for over-the-counter medications do not. The painkillers available over-the-counter, for example, can cause dangerous intestinal bleeding, yet you'd never know this from the TV advertisements for them.

• *Generally confusing the issue.* Many diagnoses carry with them a whole bag of real or perceived consequences, which usually have totally different implications. In the case of PMS, the real issue was the small percentage of women who suffered severe mood changes, not the larger percentage who suffered the bloating that the company's drug was purported to fix.

One of the most common examples of fuzzy thinking is failing to distinguish between treatments aimed at eliminating symptoms from those aimed at preventing long-term consequences. Both doctors and patients should be clear about this distinction, because the two situations call for completely different actions. If the drug or treatment is prescribed for relief of symptoms and patients end up feeling worse than when they're not taking the treatment, they should stop the drug. If the treatment is supposed to prevent long-term consequences, then patients may accept feeling worse (and then again they might not), but they should ask whether studies have been done to show that the treatment really does work and how strong the effect is.

Fibrocystic breast disease, for example, may or may not be painful, and it may or may not be (but in the vast majority of women is not) a risk factor for the development of breast cancer. The two consequences are entirely different and demand entirely different treatment strategies. If the condition leads to breast cancer and curing the fibrocystic condition will lower the risk of breast cancer, then all women with the condition ought to consider treatment. If it is simply a question of relieving pain, only those women experiencing pain bad enough to want to do something about it ought to consider treatment—and if the side effects are worse than the disease, they shouldn't hesitate to stop treatment.

Using jargon always helps confuse things, too. When the *New York Times Magazine* ran an article about treating normally short children with growth hormone, Barry Sherman, the vice president for Medical Affairs of Genentech, which makes the hormone, wrote in indignantly. Contrary to the impression given in the article, he explained, the hormone was developed first to treat children with insufficient growth hormone. He then went on to say, however, that the challenge confronting the scientific community is to understand the cause of shortness in those children who do not lack growth hormone. "While some call these children normal," he wrote, "others believe that there is a biochemical cause of their statural deficit that may be treatable with growth hormone."

In one fuzzy sentence, he has managed to pack a triple disease-mongering whammy. First of all, he implies that there is some reason to consider that these children aren't normal. Second, he uses the term *statural deficit*, which states quite clearly that these children are "deficient." Finally, he implies that there is a biochemical cause. Undoubtedly there is—for most it's probably in the genes they inherited from their parents, just as there is a biochemical cause for red hair, blue eyes, and tallness—but to proceed from there to imply that treatment is required is undoubtedly of greater benefit to Genentech than to the children.

• *Drawing an analogy between the disease you are promoting and one that is of unquestioned severity.* Menopause, for example, is often compared with diabetes, to emphasize (for those who want to sell estrogens) the relative lack of estrogen a woman produces after menopause. There are several problems here: a person with severe diabetes dies without insulin, whereas a menopausal woman does not die without estrogen treatment and, in fact, untreated, lives longer than the average man. Since all women undergo menopause, it can be considered a normal state, while severe diabetes affects only a small percentage of the population, who are definitely at a biological disadvantage if untreated. Similarly, many of those mongering Lyme disease have compared it with AIDS, even though the only thing the two seem to have in common is that they are newly recognized infectious diseases getting a lot of publicity. Lyme disease is not as severe, is not as widespread, and is curable.

• *Defining a disease as a deficiency disease or disease of hormonal imbalance.* Defining a disease this way sets the stage for drug treatment. While there are a few clear-cut deficiency diseases, in many of the conditions being promoted this way, not enough is known about normal biology to know whether someone is, in fact, deficient or simply a variant of normal.

• *Getting the right spin doctors.* Unfortunately for the organizers of the PMS meeting, they failed to use this important disease-mongering tactic. As we saw in the last chapter, there is a considerable difference of opinion among doctors of good faith as to when a condition should be diagnosed. It is only natural, then, that pharmaceutical companies, which put up much of the money for continuing medical education and definitely for press seminars, are more likely to give the money to doctors who will argue for a level of diagnosis that best serves their interests. The organizers of the PMS meeting asked the speakers to mention spironolactone by name, but most of them refused, and several made it plain in their presentations that bloating wasn't the issue and that treatment with diuretics was in most cases beside the point. If the organizers had been more careful about their spin doctors, the gauche disease-mongering tactics of the plant would not have been so apparent.

• *Framing the issues in a particular way.* One pharmaceutical company, for example, convened a press conference in Washington with the purpose of examining the costs of hypertension therapy. There are several potential approaches to cutting the costs of hypertension therapy, one of which is by defining hypertension at that level where treatment has been shown to be beneficial, which is somewhat higher than that currently used by many doctors. This, of course, would lower the number of people requiring hypertension therapy.

Indeed, the conference announcement said that it was about two recent studies, and I assumed one of them would be a large Medical Research Council Study in England that had shown that women with slightly raised blood pressure actually had a higher death rate under treatment than those not treated; another recent study showed that about one-fourth of people under treatment could be taken off the treatment and their blood pressure would remain normal. Certainly both these studies had important implications for the costs of hypertension therapy. But these studies were not brought up at all in the main body of the press conference. Instead, the speakers insisted that hypertension should be treated with cheaper drugs, and it just so happened that the company that was paying for the luncheon press conference made a diuretic, one of those cheaper drugs.

In the question-and-answer session I brought up the other studies, and one of the panelists immediately started nodding his head in vigorous agreement. After the conference he approached to tell me he was very glad I had brought up those issues because he hadn't been very happy with the general spin of the press conference but didn't feel he could say anything because he was the guest of the organizers.

• *Crying malpractice.* At a recent meeting on menopause, someone got up and said that not to treat menopausal women with hormones should be considered malpractice. Malpractice is one of those words that send chills up a doctor's spine, and the message was relayed by one of the doctors attending to a menopausal patient she saw soon afterward. Of course anyone can sue anybody for malpractice in this country and perhaps, with a clever lawyer, can win. But since hormone therapy of the menopause can cause one disease (endometrial cancer), protects against another (osteoporosis), increases the risk of another (breast cancer), and may protect against a fourth (heart disease), a doctor could get sued for either prescribing or not prescribing. A recent consensus conference at the National Institutes of Health recommended hormone therapy only in women who'd had a hysterectomy. (The problem with this, as we'll see in chapter 13, is that doctors are now recommending hysterectomy so that they can give hormone therapy in the menopause.)

• *Choosing a particularly pathetic patient who purportedly has the disease.* Leonard Sigal, M.D., Director of the Lyme Disease Center at the Robert Wood Johnson Medical School in New Brunswick, New Jersey, suggested this tactic, often used in diseases such as Lyme where overdiagnosis is rampant. Such patients often don't have Lyme disease at all, because Lyme nearly always can be cured by antibiotics. But a doctor who publicly states that these patients don't have Lyme disease will be seen as unsympathetic, as someone who is questioning the patients' suffering. If the doctor has not seen the patients' records, he or she cannot be certain that the patients do not have the disease, and if the doctor has seen the records, to cite them would be a violation of the patients' privacy.

• *Selective use of statistics to exaggerate the benefits of treatment.* Jonathan Cole, writing in *Columbia* magazine, shows how use of one statistic will tend to show a great benefit of treatment, whereas use of another will not. In a large study where 1,906 men received the cholesterol-lowering drug cholestyramine, 30 died of heart attacks over a period of ten years. In the control group of 1,900 men who didn't receive the drug, 38 died. This was a difference of 8 deaths, and one could say that this was a 24-percent reduction. But the absolute death rate was 2.0 in the control group and 1.6 in the group that received the drug, a difference that was of some statistical significance, perhaps, but not of much practical importance. While one trial of the therapy of mild hypertension purported to show that treatment reduced mortality by 20 percent, Thomas Pickering, M.D., of New York Hospital looked at the statistics in a different way and calculated that the mortality in the treated group was 6.4 percent and in the control group 7.7 percent, an actual difference of 1.3 percent.

Another way to manipulate statistics is to confuse prevalence—the number of people with a disease—with incidence—the number of people who acquire the disease in a given period of time. One pharmaceutical company promoting a vaccine for hepatitis B, for example, used figures on prevalence and presented them as incidence in an attempt to market its vaccine widely. (The ad also claimed that anyone could contract hepatitis B while, in fact, only certain groups are at significant risk.) In the case of hepatitis B, where, once acquired, the virus stays around for a number of years, prevalence figures will be much greater than incidence figures—exaggerating the degree to which one risks getting the disease.

Still another variant is confusing the lifetime risk of acquiring a disease with the risk of acquiring it in any given year. When a fund-raising volunteer from the YWCA called me for a contribution, citing the Y's support of mammography and telling me that 1-in-10 women could be expected to get breast cancer "this year," I could be somewhat forgiving of her statistical mistake, even though I knew that a woman has a one-in-nine lifetime risk of breast cancer *if she lives to the age of 110.* (The risk of a woman under 50 being diagnosed in a given year with breast cancer is about 1 in 1,000.) But the same mistake was less forgivable in the section of the *Journal of the American Medical Association* edited for medical students.

• *Using the wrong end point.* One well-known mammography study, the Breast Detection and Followup Study, was designed not to measure whether mammography worked in preventing deaths from breast cancer, but whether women could be persuaded to get mammograms. The study was deemed a success because women did come for mammograms. But the success had nothing to do with whether mammography reduced the risk of dying of breast cancer. Many studies that show that risk factors can be reduced fail to show any reduction in the diseases for which the factors predict risk—and sometimes reducing risk factors is later shown to have increased, not decreased, the death rate.

• *Promoting technology as risk-free magic.* One of the favorite selling points of doctors who advertise heavily is that whatever procedure they are touting is done by laser. Joseph C. Noreika, an ophthalmologist, explained in *Ohio Medicine* that, outside of extremely limited experimental situations, lasers are not used to remove cataracts. Yet some eye surgeons have found it advantageous to promote the image of cataract removal by laser, and patients have found it easier to deal with their surgical fantasies by relating to the perceived harmlessness of laser light. When women call to ask me about having fibroid tumors removed by laser, it's clear that many of them think they will come through the operation without a scar, not realizing that a laser is simply a high-tech knife and that even in a laser myomectomy the gynecologist will use a conventional scalpel for cutting into the abdomen, leaving a conventional scar.

• *Making treatment sound more urgent than it really is.* A purported survey about whether women would be interested in taking hormones for the prevention of osteoporosis was worded like this: "OSTEOPOROSIS is caused by thinning of the bones. Bones that become thinned by OSTEOPOROSIS are more likely to break—the HIP and the WRIST are common places for breaks. OSTEOPOROSIS may also cause back pain. These problems become more common as women get older." As Miranda Mindlin, writing in response to the article, pointed out, this letter presented the menopause in a totally negative light and detailed the horrors of osteoporosis without explaining that osteoporosis develops over a period of many years. "Surely if we want to discover perimenopausal women's views on taking hormone replacement therapy—to prevent osteoporosis or for any other purpose—we have a duty at least to provide them with information that we believe to be accurate."

In an article I wrote for *Vogue* magazine about hysterectomy, I quoted a doctor who said that she'd never seen even a large fibroid tumor damage the kidneys and that therefore a cautious approach could be taken to removing even fibroids that were quite large. I had also confirmed this with a nephrologist, or kidney specialist, although he was not quoted in the article. One doctor, who made it plain that he performed operations to remove fibroids, wrote to the editor, noting, "There is need to rush, even in an early stage if the genito-urinary tract is to be spared damage, and women not to endure unnecessary pain and stress."

• *Not correcting death rates for age.* A press release that I use in my class on medical writing, from Squibb Pharmaceuticals, which markets the drug captopril, declares: "Heart failure is a well-known killer. In the last two years, Amos and Andy co-star Freeman Gosden, Bess Truman, golfer Dutch Harrison, John Cardinal Cody, bacteriologist Rene Dubos, historian Will Durant, and critic Bosley Crowther died from heart failure." What it fails to mention is that Gosden was 83, Truman 97, Harrison 72, Cody 75, Dubos 81, Durant 96, and Crowther 75. Heart failure may be a significant cause of death, but at least in these people it doesn't seem to be a significant cause of "premature" death.

• *Taking a common symptom that could mean anything and making it sound as if it is a sign of a serious disease.* It's true that most symptoms are pretty nonspecific: if you're tired, it can mean anything from depression to a hard day at the office to cancer, so it's not, strictly speaking, dishonest to say that if you're tired, it may be cancer—it's just highly misleading. A letter to science writers and editors begins: "Maybe you have been feeling a little tired and drowsy lately. You have noticed some tenderness above the waist, perhaps a little nausea and your eyes look a bit blood-shot or sort of yellow. Oh well, just too much work, a little indigestion, too many drinks, or too much TV. These could be symptoms of liver disease." The writer, herself a sufferer from liver disease, undoubtedly wanted to get to those people like herself who did have liver disease and was willing to dismiss the fact that indeed these symptoms might be due to too much work, a little indigestion, too much TV, or too many drinks, particularly the last in the case of her fellow journalists.

Or consider this press release from Baylor College of Medicine: "Many people ignore a sore throat or a sore on their lips, mouth, gums, or tongue for a couple of weeks or longer, popping lozenges or applying medication in hopes that it will soon go away. Sometimes such a delay can have serious medical consequences. Dr. Bobby R. Alford, a head and neck surgeon at Baylor College of Medicine in Houston, views such seemingly minor conditions as possible signs of head and neck cancer—a relatively unpublicized but easily detected medical threat." Perhaps a significant delay would be important, but by implying that a two-week delay may have serious consequences, this release may send a lot of people to their doctors unnecessarily.

Psychiatrist Aaron Beck of the University of Pennsylvania, one of the fathers of cognitive therapy, suggests that the distress of the pathologically anxious arises from a combination of one or more of the following four errors: (1) overestimating the probability of a feared event, (2) overestimating the severity of the feared event, (3) underestimating coping resources (what you can do about it), and (4) underestimating rescue factors (what other people can do to help you). The gist of disease mongering lies in the first three. As to the fourth: disease-mongers *overestimate* their power to help you.

Disease-mongers, then, work to make the rest of us feel pathologically anxious, so that we'll buy their message. The chapters in Part Two offer specific examples of how they do this for specific types of problems.

Part Two

Case Studies

Chapter 6

Aches and Pains

Becoming a Patient

KNOCK: Are there many people with rheumatism in the area?
DOCTEUR PARPALAID: My dear colleague, there are nothing *but* people with rheumatism.
KNOCK: Very interesting.
DOCTEUR PARPALAID: Yes, for people who want to study rheumatism.
KNOCK, softly: I was thinking of the clients.
DOCTEUR PARPALAID: Oh! Not for that. People here would no more go to a doctor for rheumatism than go to the priest to cry.
KNOCK: But . . . that's annoying.
—Jules Romains, *Knock*

One recent hot summer's day, I was cooling off in a medical library by looking through the various journals. In those few hours, I came across a number of articles about the side effects of a group of painkilling drugs known as NSAIDs—short for nonsteroidal anti-inflammatory drugs—and sometimes referred to as prostaglandin inhibitors. The drugs are used to treat everything from rheumatoid arthritis to menstrual cramps. The side effects include everything from fatal bleeding ulcers to meningitis and are relatively common: in England, one-fourth of all adverse side effects reported from drugs are due to NSAIDs, and in the United States NSAIDs are held to cause 2,600 deaths and 20,000 hospitalizations each year in rheumatoid arthritis patients alone. In addition, people who use NSAIDs are nearly five times more likely to die of peptic ulcer disease than those who don't.

No one was calling for these drugs to be taken off the market, or indeed even made for prescription only, since they are very effective painkillers and the diseases for which they are used, such as rheumatoid arthritis, are often very painful. But the facts were nonetheless sobering.

When I went home that evening, I turned on my TV and immediately got this message: "Since most painkillers advertise they contain the same painkiller as Motrin, shouldn't you be using Motrin?" The pain killer in Motrin is, as you may have guessed, one of those NSAIDs I'd just been reading about, and there was no mention in the commercial that there was *any* risk—a classic example of minimizing the risks of treatment.

But this ad was less pernicious than some, since it at least advertised the painkiller for the use for which it is effective, that is, relieving pain. One pharmaceutical company told physicians that NSAIDs actually played a role in halting arthritis by protecting the joints—until the FDA made it stop for lack of evidence. While some NSAIDs may be less hard on the stomach than others, their promotion as remedies for stomach upset is totally unjustified, since *all* of them *damage* the stomach.

The pharmaceutical industry offers its own solution to this stomach damage: rather than calling for more restraint in prescribing NSAIDs and more vigilance in watching for side effects, it markets another drug, misoprostol, which is supposed to protect the stomach. But there's not a lot of evidence that it does, and at a cost of about $80 a month it adds significantly to the costs of therapy. While misoprostol does have *an* effect on the stomach lining that can be seen when the stomach tissues are examined, says Nortin M. Hadler, M.D., a professor of medicine and microbiology/immunology at the University of North Carolina School of Medicine in Chapel Hill, "it offers no relief from NSAID-associated symptoms and adds its own assortment of known acute and unknown long-term toxicities. And there are no data that it abrogates [lowers] the risk of significant bleeding or other gastrointestinal catastrophe."

All of us have aches and pains all the time, and if we forget about them, they usually go away. But if we happen to turn on the TV, we may be reminded of our pain and think about it more often. If we read the newspaper, we may be told that it's possibly the sign of something serious and that we should seek medical care. If we do see a doctor, he or she may organize our pains into a "disease," making it harder for us to forget about them. If we see a surgeon, the surgeon is likely to see them as a mechanical problem—a "ruptured" disk or a nerve being rubbed the wrong way—amenable to "fixing." We undergo surgery, but the pain is still there, even though the surgeon may consider the operation a success.

Michael Cherington, M.D., of the University of Colorado, cites the example of a 27-year-old woman who had progressive aching discomfort in her left arm and numbness and coldness in the fourth and fifth fingers. She was diagnosed as having "thoracic outlet syndrome," the disease discussed in chapter 3 for which a poorly tested test was used in the diagnosis for years. She had a rib removed, and following the operation she initially improved. But a few days later her arm began to feel numb and tingle. In addition, her hand and shoulder gave a burning sensation. More than a year later, her hand was extremely cold, she sweated a lot, she was pale, and her skin was extremely sensitive. This woman's minor problem had been made worse by her diagnosis and treatment.

THE PREVALENCE OF SYMPTOMS— AND HOW WE INTERPRET THEM

When people are asked if they've had various symptoms within the past week, two weeks, or six months, an enormous percentage report that they've experienced some sort of ache or pain. One recent survey, for example, in which adults were asked about their present complaints found the following:

Symptom	% Men Reporting	% Women Reporting
Headaches	39	56
Easily fatigued	33	46
Indigestion	26	29

Symptom	% Men Reporting	% Women Reporting
Cough	34	21
Constipation	18	34
Dizziness	16	29
Shortness of breath	25	22

Other studies find essentially the same thing, with slightly different numbers.

When older adults were asked about complaints they had experienced the day before, 65 percent reported fatigue or weakness and being unsteady on their feet, and 63 percent reported pain. Fifty-five percent reported worries and 43 percent upsets.

Three of every four people have symptoms in any given month, for which they take some definable action such as medication, bed rest, consulting a physician, and limiting activity. In addition, most of us experience many other symptoms, which we regard as trivial and ignore.

Disease-mongers try to convince us that such symptoms could be a sign of serious disease, and they are partially right: the symptoms sometimes are serious. But as a recent editorial by Richard Mayou in the *British Medical Journal* put it, many complaints of abdominal pain, dyspepsia, headache, backache, joint pain, chest pain, palpitations, and fatigue fall into the category of physical symptoms that cannot be traced to anything physiologically wrong in the body. While it's probably wise to consult a doctor who knows you if such symptoms are persistent, it's probably unwise to continue the search for a diagnosis if the doctor doesn't immediately come up with one. "Follow-up studies have repeatedly shown that if an initial assessment does not suggest a serious underlying physical cause, then eventually uncovering one is extremely unlikely."

Our own tolerances for such symptoms vary widely; the same person who will be blithely unaware of stomach pains one month may experience them the next. Pain is a highly subjective phenomenon, which may or may not be related to anything the doctor can see. One problem with hypochondriacs, says Arthur Barsky, M.D., a psychiatrist at Massachusetts General Hospital in Boston, is that they tend to feel bodily sensations of all sorts more intensely and tend to interpret them as disturbing. Hypochondriacs, he explained, have completely unrealistic views of good health, so they see any bodily discomfort, from a bloody nose or cramp to feeling dizzy, as a symptom. Most of us are not full-fledged hypochrondriacs, but when we read an article telling us that dizziness may be the first sign of a brain tumor, we'll probably become much more aware of any dizziness that might have been there all the time and start to worry about it.

Whether these symptoms become so apparent that we decide, in the words of Dr. Hadler, to "become a patient" will depend upon a variety of factors that may have little to do with the underlying "disease." The stomach pains this month may well be more intense than they were last month, and we tend to be bothered more by new symptoms than by symptoms that have become familiar to us. Dr. William Whitehead, an associate professor of medical psychology at Johns Hopkins University School of Medicine, has found that "as adults, we tend to pay more attention to the somatic complaints our parents paid attention to when we were young." But two other factors play an important role. One is stress: people under stress are more likely to become patients. Second, information—for example, in TV commercials, newspaper articles, or subway posters—also plays a role in making us patients. Such information influences how we interpret our symptoms and what type of specialist we may see, and the specialist we see will often determine our diagnosis.

James Pennebaker, Ph.D., author of *The Psychology of Physical Symptoms*, showed how stress and information interact to shape our perceptions of symptoms. He and his coworkers asked students either to walk or to run in place for two minutes and then escorted them into an adjacent room to complete a symptom checklist. Half the subjects were casually told, "As you know, this is the time of year when we are surrounded by flu and other illness-producing organisms." The greatest number of symptoms were reported by those subjects who ran rather than walked (in other words, were more stressed) *and* who were given the casual clue about flu, and not surprisingly the symptoms they reported were those usually associated with flu. Dr. Pennebaker thinks that the reason there haven't been more experiments of this type is that the power of suggestion on experiencing symptoms is "so easy to show. We all know people are very susceptible to suggestion."

More recent work by Dr. Pennebaker shows that women may be more susceptible to suggestions because they are less skilled at reading their internal body clues than are men, perhaps because women experience so many changes over the course of the menstrual cycle.

One of the best examples of the power of suggestion on developing, or at least recognizing, symptoms is the fact that approximately 70 percent of medical students begin to develop symptoms of the diseases they are studying. Medical sociologist David Mechanic, Ph.D., then of the University of Wisconsin in Madison, wrote that it's difficult to pinpoint the relative role of the information medical students are getting, since they are typically under quite a bit of stress, and stress also leads to more symptoms. But students in general are also typically under stress and don't appear to have such dramatic and widespread symptoms. "It seems reasonable to suspect that the medical student's access to more detailed medical information contributes greatly to the attribution process."

Dr. Mechanic went on: "The exposure to specific knowledge about disease provides the students with a new framework for identifying and giving meaning to previously neglected bodily feelings. Diffuse and ambiguous symptoms regarded as normal in the past may be interpreted according to newly acquired knowledge of disease."

Medical writers, too, go through this process of getting the diseases they write about. I remember once doing an article on autistic children, reading the list of symptoms, and deciding that perhaps I had been one myself, despite a childhood that included a good academic record, presidency of several clubs, and normal relationships with friends and family! While I had never heard of thoracic outlet syndrome before I started researching this book, I began to feel aching in my right arm about the time I started writing this chapter.

Most medical students (and most medical writers) eventually stop believing that every symptom must be the sign of a serious disease. Dr. Mechanic suggests that while reassurance from a physician on the faculty may help, further understanding of diagnostics may help students understand how they misattributed their symptoms at first. My own medical writer's symptoms tended to go away after I went to the doctor a time or two complaining of fatigue or a pain in my side, and I realized that I was being treated as a hypochondriac. I also realized that unless something was wrong that the doctor could either *measure* or see, there was no way I would be taken seriously. I then began coping with my symptoms in other ways, usually by first trying to forget about them. I learned that my stomach pains, for which the doctor had prescribed a combination tranquilizer/stomach medicine that made me quite unable to work, could be better handled by reducing the stress in my life.

However, my own symptoms probably also ended when I became aware of the dangers of diagnostic tests and unnecessary treatment, and I suspect this plays a role in medical students' diseases, too. The medically sophisticated soon learn that there is a downside to testing and treatment, and when we start adding up all the bad things that can happen with treatment, we often decide that it is probably safer to try to forget about the disease, at least until we have more definite and measurable signs. One doctor, for example, who had been ordering MRI (magnetic resonance imaging) scans of the brain for many of his own patients, found that he himself had been noticing strange sensations on the side of his head. But after undergoing an MRI himself, which he found extremely unpleasant and which didn't turn up any abnormality, he wrote in a letter to *Annals of Internal Medicine*, "I still get those sensations on my head, but you will not catch me complaining."

As Dr. Mechanic put it, "Psychologic survival generally depends on the ability of people to protect themselves from anxieties and fears involving low-risk occurrences to which all persons are exposed, or dangers that they are powerless to prevent." It is precisely such anxieties and fears that disease-mongers play upon. Because of the deficiencies in the way we get medical information from the media and often from our doctors, many laypeople remain permanently in the first stage of the medical student's disease, with a heightened sensitivity to bodily sensations but without understanding the dangers of overdiagnosis and treatment.

While it may be frustrating if your doctor clearly thinks you are wasting his or her time because you have no "disease," it may be worse to find one who validates your role as patient, particularly if, like Knock, this doctor intends to keep you a patient for his or her own good. Most commonly, you're probably going to find a doctor who simply starts ordering a round of tests to "rule out" disease, but, as we have seen in chapter 3, the tests can cause a whole new set of problems. The doctor who keeps you as a patient for his or her own good will probably be able to rationalize that you need a sympathetic shoulder to cry on, and the way to show sympathy is to give you a diagnosis, which will give you "validation" of your suffering as well as possible insurance coverage for your medical visits.

HOW DOCTORS ORGANIZE ACHES AND PAINS

Doctors "organize" the aches and pains that are so widespread into "diseases," which then take on a life of their own, leading to "treatments of choice," specific payments, and, for aches and pains possibly acquired in the workplace, claims for worker's compensation. The following are some of the ways aches and pains get organized into diseases.

Fibrositis

Suppose that your muscles ache. If you present these symptoms to a doctor, the doctor may call them "fibrositis." Fibrositis is one of those diagnoses made by the Chinese restaurant menu: there are "obligatory" criteria, "major" criteria, and "minor" criteria listed. Making the diagnosis is rather like assembling a poker hand: to qualify for the diagnosis, you must have the obligatory and major criteria plus three minor critera; or the obligatory critera, three tender points, and five minor criteria. However, it should be noted that two of the obligatory criteria are basically "rule-out" criteria: there must be no underlying cause, and laboratory tests must be normal. The one remaining obligatory criterion is that there is generalized musculoskeletal aching pain and/or stiffness of at least three months' duration. Ultimately, then, fibrositis means that you've been aching or stiff for at least three months, and no one has a clue as to why.

Such symptoms are exceedingly common. If you ask patients in a general medical clinic about their symptoms, nearly 10 percent meet the criteria for fibrositis. If you examine 100 well men and 100 well women serving in the military, half demonstrate one or more typical "trigger points." While it is unclear what drives people with such symptoms to report them to a physician, once they do—and not before—they begin to develop generalized rheumatism.

As a part of the exercise of diagnosis, Dr. Hadler points out, the physician will restructure the patient's perceptions so that the patient will soon start to focus upon all sorts of symptoms that they usually hadn't been aware of before. The patient now has new language and new associations. All of a sudden, he or she becomes acutely aware of previously unfamiliar terms such as vascular lability of the digits, trigger points, and tender points and begins to focus on duration of stiffness, sleep pattern, and fatigue. Such a patient, says Dr. Hadler, leaves the office with a dramatically, irretrievably altered illness.

"Any attempt to cope with new symptoms . . . is thwarted. All symptoms, new and old, are remembered, considered, even recorded under the banner of the diagnostic exercise. The process must be identified, labeled, treated, and banished." Generalized rheumatism, sometimes called fibrositis, is not a diagnosis, Dr. Hadler claims, but a process of instruction in illness behavior.

Repetitive Strain Injury and Tendinitis

There are other ways to organize aches and pains into "diseases" that are questionable and may lead to more harm than good. One is repetitive strain injury (RSI), which some say is linked to workplace trauma; again, the symptoms of this disease are extremely common, even in people who do not have work that requires repetitive strain. Dr. Hadler points out that over 25 percent of those people who work in tasks requiring the least force and repetitiveness experience arm pain occurring more than once or lasting more than one week in the previous two years. Yet there's no evidence that repetitive tasks cause irreversible damage to the joints. A study from Ann Arbor, Michigan, found that workers who had highly forceful and repetitive tasks were more likely to have wrist tenderness upon examination. This is all that is meant by "tendinitis," Dr. Hadler says. "'Wrist soreness' would be a far more appropriate clinical label. . . . We're all accustomed to such episodes. Typically, we seldom even tell our doctor."

If a worker does take this to worker's compensation, then he or she may lose the right to refuse treatment, and may be subjected to surgery, which probably isn't going to help, particularly if the person has to go back to doing the same task. "What possesses surgeons to intervene as if desperate on behalf of these fearful, anxious, 'injured' workers when the same surgeons would exercise far more caution in other settings?" asks Dr. Hadler. Workplaces that give rise to epidemics of repetitive strain disorder are usually angry, unstable, unpleasant, and unappealing work environments, he says. "Nonetheless, someone trustworthy needs to articulate a perspective in these settings that allows the workers to maintain control of their medical destiny. Causing them to feel so much alarm, in the absence of substantive evidence, is irresponsible and unconscionable."

Worker's compensation plays its own role in making patients, since in the absence of measurable injury a patient must prove that he or she is hurting. Now the worker probably is hurting, but the best way to heal the hurt may be to try to forget about it and perhaps change the workplace task. But once an action is taken in worker's compensation, the worker-patient has two conflicting interests. To forget about the hurt and try to heal may be best for the worker's health, but to concentrate on the hurt and try to prove its existence may result in a compensation payment.

Even physicians who are more willing to accept the concept of repetitive strain injury nonetheless agree with Dr. Hadler that operations are usually not the answer; the answer may be to remove the worker from the particular job that is causing the problems. Martin G. Cherniack, M.D., agrees: "The majority of vibration-exposed workers will not benefit from surgery and, in any case, symptoms, if relieved, will usually recur following return to work." The temptation to operate, he cautions, "must be disregarded because of the poor likelihood of success." Dr. Cherniack points out that another aspect of worker's compensation leads to unhelpful surgery. After surgery, it is up to the surgeon to judge how much the arm or leg is still not functioning normally, known as the residual deficit, so that the worker can receive a lump sum payment. There's no particular way to measure this, and surgeons aren't likely to want to admit that there's still a 40 percent deficit after they have done their best. So surgeons commonly give a figure of 3 to 4 percent, even if the real deficit is much greater than that. "If the surgeons admitted to a 40 percent deficit after surgery, insurance companies wouldn't be willing to pay for the surgery," Dr. Cherniack points out.

Back Pain

Jerry J. Jasinowksi, president of the National Association of Manufacturers, wrote in the *New York Times* that a painful back sent him to top medical specialists in Washington and New York. "One doctor rated the injury an 8 on a scale of 1 to 10 and recommended immediate surgery. The other rated it a 2 and suggested plenty of rest and physical therapy. I opted for the latter and am in fine physical shape today."

The two doctors Jasinowksi saw held two very different ways of organizing his back pain into a "disease." The first likely saw it as resulting from an injury and described it in terms of a herniated or "ruptured" disk. The second saw it as similar to headache: a pain that would eventually go away on its own.

Back pain is inordinately common, with over half of us experiencing it for at least a week out of every six weeks, but only 0.3 percent of the population going on to become back pain patients. Dr. Hadler points out that prior to 1934, back pain was never seen as being due to an injury. In that year, two surgeons published several cases of backache in which they found an associated herniation. "Not only did they infer a causal role for herniation . . . in the pathogenesis of backache, they labeled the process 'rupture.'"

Rupture, Dr. Hadler points out, "is a highly evocative term; it describes something being broken or burst! When a patient is told he 'ruptured his disk,' he envisions major anatomic disruption."

The use of the term rupture had other major consequences. It led to surgical "solutions." It led worker's compensation administrators to compensate, because the term rupture seemed to imply an injury. "To this day, in almost every workers' compensation jurisdiction, if a worker's backache is certified by a physician to result from a ruptured disk, the worker will be compensated." The chief complaint of backache sufferers, Dr. Hadler points out, became and remains, "I injured my back," rather than "Oh, my aching back."

The rub is that while it's true that most patients suffering back pain can be found to have "ruptured" disks, once doctors started examining patients who didn't have back pain, they found "ruptured" disks, too. By midlife 30 to 40 percent of people have them, and in the 60 to 70 age range, 70 to 80 percent of people have a "ruptured" disk, whether or not they feel, or indeed ever felt, pain. This, of course, calls into question just what role the ruptured disk plays in causing the backache as well as whether surgery can lessen that pain. It's true the pain may disappear after surgery, but studies have shown that it will disappear just as rapidly without surgery, except possibly in cases where the back pain is associated with leg pain.

New York *Newsday* columnist Marty Goldensohn, for example, found that even though his CT-scan showed compression at two vertebrae, he was cured not by an operation, but by finding a doctor who reorganized the way he saw his disease. The doctor, who Goldensohn refers to as Dr. Spine, explained to Goldensohn that muscles go into spasm to distract you from your anger. "As soon as you hear that, you get so embarrassed you never have another episode."

Goldensohn found the explanation so effective that he began persuading all his friends to see Dr. Spine. One, a pianist who was scheduled for back surgery in three days, insisted: "Not me. I've ruptured a disk. My CT-Scan shows vertebral compression at L-4,L-5." Goldensohn finally persuaded the friend not to have surgery but to have an exam and two lectures from Dr. Spine.

After that, his friend was able to forgo surgery and play Rachmaninoff without a twinge.

Thoracic Outlet Syndrome

Thoracic outlet syndrome, as we've already mentioned, (see pages 42–43) is a label given to patients with symptoms in the arm such as weakness and tingling and sometimes wasting of the hand and forearm muscles. Sometimes this syndrome is due to pressure on the blood vessels, which is easy to document with specific tests. Occasionally, probably one case in a million, the syndrome is a classic neurogenic thoracic outlet syndrome (TOS), where an extra rib holds a fibrous band that grates against the nerve that leads to the arm, causing aches and weakness.

But 85 percent of people diagnosed with "neurogenic" thoracic outlet syndrome don't have the extra rib and in fact have no objective signs of the syndrome. The subjective symptoms, usually weakness and perhaps tingling in the arm, are the same, but there is little or no wasting of the hand and forearm muscles. While these patients are treated by taking out a normal rib, this operation is not always successful. "Many patients with symptoms attributed to nonspecific neurogenic TOS can be relieved without resection of the first rib," wrote Drs. Albert C. Cuetter and David M. Bartoszek, of the William Beaumont Army Medical Center in El Paso, Texas. They suggest that if patients are given this diagnosis, they should make sure that their pains aren't really due to another condition, such as carpal tunnel syndrome, before they have their rib removed.

In an article titled "Surgery for Thoracic Outlet Syndrome May Be Hazardous for Your Health," Dr. Michael Cherington and his co-authors reported five patients who had minor problems that were diagnosed as TOS who developed worse problems after their surgery. One 28-year-old woman, for example, had her rib removed and found afterward she had profound weakness in her right arm, with severe weakness in the hand. She also didn't have much sensation in her hand and was unable to return to work.

Dr. Cherington notes that many patients of the so-called syndrome continue to have symptoms after their surgery, even though their surgery has been called a success. "I believe there are many of us who think that surgery for thoracic outlet syndrome is hazardous for patients and should be undertaken rarely if at all." He also points out that surgery for TOS is mostly a hazard for patients with health insurance: of 209 TOS patients treated in Colorado in 1989, 179 had surgical treatment, and 30 were treated conservatively. Of the surgical patients, 67 percent had health insurance, and 27 percent had worker's compensation; only 3 percent paid for the operation themselves, and another 3 percent had Medicaid. "Patients who do not have private insurance or worker's compensation coverage almost never undergo surgery," concluded Dr. Cherington.

Carpal Tunnel Syndrome

The diagnosis of carpal tunnel syndrome is another that should always be taken with a grain of salt, particularly if the doctor recommends surgery. Carpal tunnel syndrome is caused when one of the nerves passing through the fibrous bridge in the wrist, known as the carpal tunnel, is compressed, leading to pins-and-needles, numbness, or pain in the fingers. Dr. Cherniak points out that the diagnosis of carpal tunnel syndrome is given for about seven or eight different processes, of which two may have a surgical solution. While surgery will usually relieve symptoms, says Dr. Dean S. Louis of the University of Michigan Hospitals, the symptoms will begin again once the worker finds himself doing the same job. "In this situation, the people who receive the most benefit from the scenario are the lawyer, and . . . the hand surgeon. Surgical thinking has promoted the idea that the carpal tunnel syndrome is a surgical disease."

"After the resolution of symptoms during the early phase, the worker is left in the unenviable position of not being able to pursue the most reasonable alternative—to seek other employment or to accept a less hand-intensive job in his current workplace. To seek other employment might deny the possibility of receiving worker's compensation."

The bottom line seems to be that we should watch out for surgeons who recommend immediate surgery for our aches and pains. We should seek out second opinions not from other surgeons, but from nonsurgeons such as rheumatologists or neurologists, who not only have no financial reason to recommend surgery but who also may organize the aches and pains into the model of a different disease—one that doesn't lend itself to a surgical solution.

But we should also beware those who would tell us we have a "disease" that only they can cure, even without surgery. Most often, when the problem is aches and pains, the goal should be to make your symptoms bearable until your body can heal itself: a healing that is usually long-lasting, cheap, effective, and much less fraught with risk than many of the treatments being mongered.

Chapter 7

Lyme Disease and "Lime" Disease

Knock: It demonstrates, clear as day, with the aid of case histories, that you can walk around plump, with a rosy tongue, an excellent appetite, and have in all the folds of your body trillions of bacteria of the utmost virulence capable of infecting the whole county. Strong in theory and in experience, I have the right to suspect the first person who comes to be a carrier. You, for example, absolutely nothing proves to me that you're not one.
—Jules Romains, *Knock*

In the mid-1970s two women living in the towns of Lyme and Old Lyme, Connecticut, started to call attention to the epidemic of swollen and painful joints and other symptoms among their family and friends. The women persisted until they got a young doctor from Yale University, Dr. Allen Steere, interested in the mini-epidemic. The disease eventually became known as Lyme disease, even though it later turned out that European doctors had recognized various aspects of it during the first quarter of this century. In 1982, the microorganism that caused it, transmitted by ticks that lived on deer and mice, was named *Borrelia burgdorferi*.

At least one of the women persisted in her quest because she couldn't accept the fact that her daughter had been diagnosed with juvenile rheumatoid arthritis, a disease for which there is no cure and that can leave its sufferers crippled. She was right to try to find another explanation, since the Lyme disease that her daughter really had and that she helped to discover is usually quite easily cured with antibiotics. But, ironically, a decade after the initial cases were identified, an epidemic fear of Lyme disease was gripping the Northeast, upper Midwest, and other parts of the country. Many people who had never heard of juvenile rheumatoid arthritis were altering their lives in sometimes bizarre ways to avoid Lyme disease. Rather than taking the simple precautions of tucking their pant legs into their socks and showering after being outdoors, people were avoiding the outdoors altogether; rather than simply being aware of the symptoms of Lyme disease they were getting antibiotics if they so much as found a tick crawling on them; and rather than seeing their doctors if they developed symptoms, some were even going to Mexico for injections of live malaria to cure their so-called Lyme disease—even though malaria is a much more serious disease than Lyme. What had in fact transformed this occasionally serious, yet almost always curable, disease into one that people were comparing with AIDS?

"I really don't understand," says Leonard H. Sigal, M.D., Director of the Lyme Disease Center at Robert Wood Johnson Medical School in New Brunswick, New Jersey. "I'm really mystified by the degree of anxiety. Furthermore," he said, "I consider it an abomination that people can compare a 100 percent fatal disorder with a disease which is for the most part easily treated and cured and almost certainly has resulted in fewer than 10 fatalities around the world."

THE PLAYERS

No one player seems to be totally responsible for what doctors by the early 1990s were variously referring to as "Lime" disease, Lyme anxiety, or *Borreliosis neurosis*. Certainly it had something to do with the fact that Americans have always felt the natural environment to be fraught with hazards, and a bacterium harbored by ticks that live on deer or mice gave us a triple whammy from the environment. Much more than our European cousins, we Americans have a collective national phobia about germs and very little understanding of the considerable defenses that a healthy body naturally mobilizes against them. Playing on this long-standing fear were manufacturers of tick repellant, who broadcast scary advertisements and made direct comparisons of Lyme disease with AIDS. The press let itself be seduced by this analogy and played its role by promoting Lyme disease as more widespread and serious than it really was. What's more, Lyme disease was "new" and by definition "news." Medical writers urged people to seek antibiotic treatment early without defining what "early" was. Many commercial tests were marketed that were neither very accurate nor capable of diagnosing the disease, since the diagnosis can be made only on the basis of symptoms. Some physicians, who have come to be known as the "Lime" doctors, played a role by using diagnostic criteria so loose that anybody who half wanted to have Lyme disease could get it without even going into the woods. People falsely diagnosed as having Lyme disease naturally did not respond to antibiotics, promoting the idea that Lyme disease was incurable.

THE FAILURE OF HEALTH EDUCATION

If blame for the widespread fear of Lyme disease is to be assigned, the first responsibility lies with the failure of health education in this country to emphasize that people are born with considerable defenses against encounters with germs of all sorts and that simply coming into contact with a germ, or an insect that might be carrying a germ, rarely results in disease. Despite my education in biochemistry and physiology and my many years as a medical journalist, it was only during a long stay as a medical reporter in Europe that I began to realize how important these defenses are. Nobody within the medical community emphasizes this fact because it's to nobody's advantage but the patient's; doctors, both orthodox and unorthodox, as well as the manufacturers of various remedies, find it all too easy to take credit for doing what the body's immune system has actually done all by itself.

In the case of Lyme disease, the body's defenses are considerable. Even if you are bitten by a tick that is infected with Borrelia burgdorferi, the tick probably has to stay on you for anywhere from 24 to 48 hours in order to transmit the bacterium, although Dr. Sigal notes that this has been shown only in animal experiments: "It's hard to get humans to let us test them for this." Even in the northeastern areas where Lyme disease is most common, "only one or two percent of tick bites will transfer the disease." While several doctors started studies to determine whether prophylactic antibiotics—giving antibiotics when the tick bite is discovered, rather than waiting for symptoms—were effective in heading off Lyme, so few patients developed Lyme disease regardless of whether or not they were given antibiotics that there weren't enough cases to obtain significant results.

Even if you do get infected, your chances of recovering fully without any treatment at all are good. A considerable number of people give a positive test for Lyme disease without any history of ever being sick. "Ten to 20 percent of people have been exposed to Lyme disease in the past, their body localized and wiped it out and they never got sick," says neurologist Michael Finkel, M.D., medical director of the Western Wisconsin Lyme Disease Center in Eau Claire. Only about 10 percent of people who do get sick with Lyme disease go on to develop chronic arthritis lasting a year or longer, even without treatment.

While medical educators have failed to provide a broad perspective on how the body can defend itself, the press might have emphasized this aspect more than it did. Instead, they emphasized the seriousness of the disease. Comparisons with syphilis were probably inevitable, since the bacterium that causes Lyme disease is the same type that causes syphilis, and the two diseases have certain features in common. But syphilis carries connotations that are unnecessarily frightening, due to its associations with tawdry sex and the fact that it was well known and fatal in the preantibiotic era.

But the comparisons didn't stop with syphilis: people went on to compare Lyme disease with AIDS. One local paper in Westchester County, for example, quoted an entomologist (shown in a picture applying tick repellant to someone's lawn) comparing Lyme disease with AIDS based on its suppression of the immune system. Ticks do produce a substance that suppresses the immune system locally. But the entomologist was quoted as saying, "The controversial question is: Can the tick really suppress our immune system completely? What parts of the immune system is it suppressing? For how long?

"The acquired immune deficiency syndrome [AIDS] suppresses the immune system to the point that it does not work at all. Lyme disease is the number two disease behind AIDS," the entomologist explained, "only because it's not considered life-threatening." The quote makes no sense if you analyze it, since it's the life-threatening nature of AIDS that makes it such a serious and feared disease. But for the casual reader, the damage is done: Lyme disease is made to appear almost as serious as AIDS.

The failure to emphasize that contact with ticks, or even a tick bite, doesn't necessarily lead to Lyme disease gave rise to a heightened sense of danger as well as a confusion as to what was meant by early treatment. Certain doctors quoted in the press added to the confusion. Dr. Joseph J. Burrascano, of East Hampton, was quoted in a Newsday article, which was otherwise well balanced, saying that "here on Long Island we figure that 80 percent of the deer ticks are infected with Lyme, and that puts every single resident at risk." The local Westchester paper urged everyone with a tick bite to start oral antibiotics while in the meantime mailing the offending tick off in an Identitick kit ($25) to a laboratory to find out whether it was carrying Lyme disease. "If the tick is not infected, that's the end of treatment. If the tick is infected, you continue the antibiotics for the full course of treatment and cure," advised the writer.

It's easy to claim that antibiotics have cured the Lyme disease that someone never had in the first place, and whether or not the Identitick test was positive, it's not whether the tick has Lyme disease that is important: it's whether you do. To have Lyme disease, by definition, you have to have symptoms. Lyme disease experts such as Drs. Daniel W. Rahn and Stephen E. Malawista, of Yale University School of Medicine, point out that there's no harm in waiting for symptoms before starting antibiotic treatment, and this in fact is what is meant by "early treatment."

OVERDIAGNOSIS

Stephen Luger, M.D., a family practitioner in Old Lyme, Connecticut, who has published several papers on Lyme disease, points out that while in most infectious diseases a positive diagnosis means that the doctor has actually isolated the offending germ, in Lyme disease the criteria are already somewhat looser because all that is required is a positive test that reveals antibody to the germ and a symptom or two that might easily be due to something else.

A lot of people with positive antibody tests don't have any disease; Dr. Sigal points out that of every 40 people who show a positive test only one actually has any evidence of disease. In addition, sending the same patient's blood to different laboratories often gives very different results. One group sent blood samples from 22 persons to four different laboratories. Eight were positive at all four laboratories, but all 22 were positive in at least one laboratory, implying that nearly everybody can get a positive test if he or she is persistent enough.

The word got out that the test for Lyme disease wasn't very accurate, but the press, public, and many doctors interpreted this in a way that would have been immensely pleasing to Knock. Rather than treating it as a two-edged sword (you could be either a false positive or a false negative), only the false negatives were emphasized. You could be harboring the Lyme disease bacterium even if you tested negative, and so many doctors prescribed antibiotics even to those patients who had no symptoms and who were negative.

Actually, false negatives were quite rare, due mostly to the fact that either the test was ordered too soon or antibiotics were prescribed too soon, therefore aborting the body's natural immune response. The greater problem with the test by far was the false positives, resulting in an inordinate number of people getting antibiotics. Dr. Sigal studied the first 100 patients seen at the Lyme Disease Center in New Brunswick and concluded that only 37 probably had either current or past Lyme disease and that about half of the courses of antibiotics they had been given had been unnecessary.

As fear of Lyme disease spread, a large number of tests were ordered. In Wisconsin, for example, where 7.5 cases of Lyme disease per 100,000 population were identified, there were 1,200 tests for every 100,000 persons, meaning that there were 160 tests for every person found to have Lyme disease. Many of the tests came out falsely positive, and with doctors telling people with negative tests that they might have Lyme disease anyway, the number of reported cases was rising precipitously, with nobody quite certain whether there really was more Lyme disease or whether people were just diagnosing more of it. While Jane Brody, the *New York Times* health columnist, had earlier written a balanced column about Lyme disease, urging people not to overreact, she couldn't resist in a 1991 column defining Lyme disease as "a tick-borne bacterial infection that is spreading faster than any other ailment except AIDS" and saying Lyme afflicted 30,000 cases last year, when, in fact, 30,000 was the total number diagnosed since the epidemic began. Two days after her column came out, the Centers for Disease Control announced that Lyme disease was leveling off at about 8,000 cases a year, perhaps after the federal government adopted a definition of the disease. In Georgia, for example, reported cases dropped from 715 in 1989 to 161 in 1990 after the state discontinued free testing and sponsored educational seminars on Lyme disease.

THE "LIME" DOCTORS

While things were confusing enough for doctors trying to do right by their patients, "Lime" doctors, as they came to be called by their colleagues, adopted extremely loose diagnostic criteria. As Drs. Daniel S. Berman and Barry D. Wenglin, of White Plains, New York, wrote in a letter to the *Annals of Internal Medicine*: "There has been a proliferation of "Lime" physicians who are making the diagnosis of Lyme disease in anybody who is interested in having the diagnosis made. Further, these physicians are prescribing regimens of oral and intravenous antibiotics lasting weeks and often months."

What was happening was that large numbers of patients complaining of vague symptoms had latched onto the diagnosis of Lyme disease and sought out a doctor who would make it, presumably validating their suffering. Dr. Burrascano, for example, said people from 32 states and 6 foreign countries have flocked to his office in East Hampton to be treated for chronic Lyme disease.

His seven telephone lines are backed up with so many calls he has stopped taking new cases. "If I could clone myself," he was quoted as saying in *Newsday*, "I could treat 1,000 patients."

Doctors who made the diagnosis of Lyme disease loosely often claim that they are more sympathetic to their patients' suffering than other doctors who refuse to make the diagnosis. But why a doctor has to give a specific diagnosis and lots of antibiotics, making considerable money in the process, to be labeled sympathetic raises the question of who is benefiting. A sympathetic doctor is one who listens, takes your complaints seriously, and when appropriate, explains that medicine doesn't have all the answers.

Usually by defining a disease loosely, many people who aren't that sick get included in the definition, adding to the numbers but diluting the seriousness of the average case. (This, as we'll see in Chapter 11, is what happens with the condition known as mitral valve prolapse.) But in Lyme disease the opposite occurred, with the wide definition including many people who, because they don't really have Lyme disease, don't respond to antibiotics. A failure to respond often resulted in a prescription for even more antibiotics. "If they don't have Lyme," says Dr. Sigal, "they don't get better on their first course of antibiotics, so they get another and another and another—it's frightening."

THE SIDE EFFECTS OF ANTIBIOTICS

Many people would consider that it's always better to give antibiotics "just in case," forgetting that antibiotics can cause considerable mischief themselves. Dr. Sigal knows of at least two girls in the New Jersey area who had to have their gallbladders removed because of inappropriate treatment with the antibiotic ceftriaxone, which creates a sludge in the gallbladder. Countless others suffered yeast infections, colitis, allergic reactions, and other well-documented side effects of antibiotics—including the fact that they can cost a lot.

A naturalist, for example, found 37 ticks on her skin a couple of days after a weekend hiking at Montauk State Park on Long Island, New York. While only one, which she was able to identify as a dog tick, had engorged, some of the others were deer ticks, and the fact that she discovered them several days after her weekend caused her to see a doctor. The doctor, who charged $125, asked her if she was allergic to penicillin, and she said no, since she had never previously had a problem with the antibiotic.

Three days later she had a rash over most of her body, and she returned to the doctor, who insisted that she get a second opinion from a dermatologist. The dermatologist charged another $125, no small sum for a free-lance naturalist who had no health insurance and earned only about $9,000 that year. The dermatologist diagnosed a drug reaction, prescribed some salves, and switched the antibiotic, telling her that the rash would soon go away. The second antibiotic, which brought her drug costs up to $60, made her feel nauseated and gave her terrible diarrhea so she took it for only 10 of the 22 days she was supposed to. The rash took three months to clear up, and she has had no symptoms of Lyme disease, even though taking an incomplete course of antibiotics was probably worse than taking none at all since it could have conferred antibiotic resistance on any germs present. "I was a healthy person going to a doctor for advice," she says of the episode, which cost her $310, a three-month rash, nausea, and diarrhea.

The saga of Lyme disease should make us all suspicious of one-disease doctors, analogies to AIDS or other undoubtedly serious diseases, and diseases reputed to be sweeping the country like wildfire. A disease is a disease by definition, and until it is defined, the diagnosis is up for grabs. The question is, Do you really want it?

Chapter 8

If You're Tired, You Have . . .

The lament of the ill, all the ill for all times, is 'why me?' St. Thomas Aquinas deprived us of the facile answer, 'fate.' There had to be a pathogenic explanation, no matter how contrived.
— Nortin M. Hadler, *Clinical Orthopaedics and Related Research,* 1987.

The title of the book caught my eye: *What Really Killed Gilda Radner?* Since I knew that Gilda Radner had written a book about her struggle with ovarian cancer, I was puzzled to see that the subtitle of the book was *Frontline Reports on the Chronic Fatigue Syndrome Epidemic.* The book's author, Neenyah Ostrom, claims that it was not ovarian cancer, but chronic fatigue syndrome, that killed Radner. A year and a half before she was diagnosed with ovarian cancer, the author points out, Radner was diagnosed as having chronic fatigue syndrome. "Did Gilda Radner die as a direct result of the government's cover-up of chronic fatigue syndrome? Were U.S. health authorities' manipulation and misrepresentation of data, phony theories, and general lack of concern for people with chronic fatigue syndrome contributing factors?"

One wonders what Gilda Radner herself would have thought of all this.

CHRONIC FATIGUE SYNDROME

The diseasing of the very common symptom of fatigue leads to this particular flip-flop of logic. Most serious diseases have fatigue as one of their symptoms, and since many diseases such as cancer are usually present long before they can be diagnosed, the fatigue often precedes the cancer diagnosis. It's an interesting *possibility* that lots of cancers result from chronic fatigue syndrome. But it's also very unlikely.

Fatigue is a symptom ripe for mongering. It's ubiquitous. Nearly anything causes it, including serious disease, normal work, viral illnesses, and depression. We'd all like to have more energy and less fatigue. There's no definition of when fatigue becomes medically significant. Fatigue is widespread and sometimes serious, and by lumping our fatigue with Gilda Radner's we can be easily convinced that our fatigue, too, is likely to be the sign of an impending death. As Dr. John Kirk, an internist who heads the Dartmouth COOP Project, a primary care research network, says, "Fatigue lends itself well to exploitation."

Americans tend to admire the person who not only can have it all, but can do it all. How many times have we read the profile of the achiever who can get up at five in the morning, jog for an hour, do a Russian lesson before work begins, and dance until midnight after it ends? We'd all *like* to be able to do this and have the vague impression that there is something wrong with us if we don't. One woman of my acquaintance, for example, told me she *used* to follow such a schedule, even though when I used to know her, she never got up before eight in the morning. A physician I interviewed about systemic lupus erythematosus, a sometimes serious disease characterized by a disorder of the immune system, defined abnormal fatigue as the inability of a woman (most lupus sufferers are women) to go out in the evening after working a full day. I was too cowed to tell him that, while I don't suffer from lupus, I couldn't go out every evening after working a full day, and I am considered by my friends as someone who goes out a lot!

People like my friend and the physician seem to have totally unrealistic ideas about how much energy is normal, how much energy they used to have, and how much energy they ought to have now. Many people, for example, often exclaim, "I don't have as much energy as I used to have. I used to be able to stay up most of the night!" What they have forgotten is that those late college nights were often followed by a day of sleeping *very* late and that it's not that they're getting more sleep these days, but that they're getting it at different times. Even if they are not overestimating the energy they used to have, says Dr. Kirk, "people think that when they're 75, they should have as much energy as when they were 40."

When people in the general population are asked about fatigue, something like 14 to 25 percent of men and 20 to 41 percent of women admit to frequent feelings of fatigue. Fatigue is one of the most common symptoms that bring patients to see the doctor, and in a recent survey of a university general practice clinic, 37 percent of patient visits involved chronic, disabling fatigue; in 59 percent of these cases no medical cause was found. While fatigue is commonly presented to doctors—indeed, it is a sign of nearly all physical and mental diseases—the medical profession has not been much help in deciding when fatigue becomes severe enough to worry about. Dr. Kirk says that for the Dartmouth COOP project's study of fatigue as a symptom, they tried to find a medically significant definition of fatigue but couldn't. "We don't have a practical definition," he says. "Each physician will have their own rule of thumb. For example, is a patient carrying out all their normal activities, with their fatigue being mostly an emotional feeling?"

Because fatigue can mean so many different diseases and is so poorly defined, it is highly susceptible to cultural interpretations, both as to when it becomes significant and what it signifies. Cultures that emphasize achievement and constantly doing things are more likely to consider fatigue pathological, and Dr. Simon Wessely, a British psychiatrist, points out that chronic fatigue syndrome surfaced in Margaret Thatcher's Britain and Ronald Reagan's America, when individual achievement—which requires a lot of energy—was being emphasized. Each country's doctors tend to have a favorite "wastebasket" diagnosis for fatigue, with German doctors likely to consider it a sign of "cardiac insufficiency"; French doctors, "spasmophilia" (a predisposition to hyperventilate, often treated with magnesium supplements); English doctors, "depression"; and American doctors, "a virus."

BACKGROUND

Syndromes characterized by chronic fatigue have been around for a long time: in the last century chronic fatigue used to be known as neurasthenia, which European doctors called "the American disease." The French psychiatrist Charcot, for example, wrote: "It is actually true that many Americans have a way of working which is peculiarly their own: once they have set themselves a task, they stick to it stubbornly for a considerable period of time which sometimes runs into years. They go to extremes, they make it a matter of pride, nothing distracts them, and after a certain time, they fall a prey to neurasthenia. After so much work their poor brain refuses to function any longer."

Since Americans have always favored microbial explanations of disease, it is not surprising that they favor viral explanations for chronic fatigue. In late 1984 and early 1985, a series of articles began linking the Epstein-Barr virus (EBV) to a chronic illness, based on what seemed to be large amounts of antibody to the EBV in persons with the syndrome. Since the EBV is known to cause infectious mononucleosis, which indeed makes people very tired, it seemed logical that perhaps some people were unable to rid the virus from their bodies, resulting in a chronic fatigue. But when the Centers for Disease Control studied the epidemic more closely, they found that the levels of antibody varied widely in persons presumed to have the disease and were usually within the normal range.

Despite this finding, which should have raised significant doubts as to whether the virus was causing the fatigue, Gary P. Holmes, of the Centers for Disease Control (CDC) in Atlanta, told a 1990 meeting on the syndrome, "The chronic [C]EBV syndrome became a popular and widespread diagnosis by early 1986."

As with so many other popular diagnoses, "the criteria used to confirm the diagnosis by individual physicians and by researchers," Dr. Holmes said, "were highly variable and often so vague as to potentially include persons who had multiple identifiable chronic diseases." For example, a study of patients diagnosed with chronic EBV by internists in Atlanta showed that the internists frequently failed to evaluate the symptoms for other possible causes. "In summary, CEBV had become a very

popular and even trendy diagnosis that was based upon laboratory tests that were nonspecific and were really not diagnostic,
many patients were not being adequately evaluated for other
possible causes of their illnesses, and the diagnostic criteria for
diagnosis varied widely from physician to physician."

Because there wasn't good evidence that the syndrome was
caused by infection with Epstein-Barr virus, researchers felt the
need to find a new name for the syndrome. Because the diagnosis
was so vague, they decided that it was necessary to agree on some
specific diagnostic criteria. In April 1986, the CDC organized an
informal working group to address these issues, and the syndrome
was renamed the chronic fatigue syndrome.

The "official" definition of chronic fatigue syndrome given
by the CDC is somewhat more precise than the definition of
fatigue itself: the person must have fatigue severe enough to
reduce daily activity by half of his or her normal routine; the
person must have had a total of 8 of 14 other symptoms, such as
fever, sore throat, painful lymph nodes, unexplained muscle
weakness, muscle pain, and prolonged fatigue after exercise, for
more than six months. In addition, all other possible causes must
already have been excluded. But here, too, there is considerable
room for subjectivity. There is still no definition of fatigue itself,
and if people seem to overestimate the amount of energy they
had in the past, as I believe most people do, reducing it by half
may still allow a person to carry out a routine that others may see
as quite normal. The other criteria include symptoms, such as
sleep disturbance and inability to concentrate, that can be highly
subjective.

Dr. Holmes admits that "the chronic fatigue syndrome remains
a vague, poorly understood illness that cannot be absolutely
diagnosed and confirmed in an individual patient."

One physician, Dr. Walter Wilson, chief of infectious diseases
at the Mayo Clinic in Rochester, Minnesota, offered some insight
as to why doctors make the diagnosis. He noted that overachieving
young adults who lead stressful lives are often affected with
chronic fatigue, and such patients pose a dilemma. "Most have
already consulted a number of doctors who had told them there
was nothing wrong. Yet they demand an explanation, if not
definitive treatment.

"They don't want to spend a lot of money flying to the Mayo, staying in a hotel and paying for meals, to hear me say there is nothing wrong with them. That is the last thing they want to hear, and you have to treat them with respect for what they are going through."

Robert Layzer, M.D., a professor of neurology at the University of California at San Francisco, points out that the CDC definition of chronic fatigue syndrome specifically excludes patients with psychiatric disease, yet this exclusion eliminates the majority of people with chronic fatigue encountered in medical practice. At the Fatigue Clinic of the University of Connecticut Health Center, 67 percent of patients had psychiatric disorders, 3 percent had medical disorders, and 25 percent didn't really meet the CDC definition because they didn't have enough of the minor criteria. Only 6 percent met the CDC definition for chronic fatigue syndrome.

One problem with most of the information that's coming out about fatigue, says Dr. Kirk, is that both chronic fatigue and chronic fatigue syndrome are probably due to a variety of causes, yet the identification of chronic fatigue syndrome tends to make people think that fatigue is due to one particular agent. Each new report that a particular virus was found in association with the "syndrome" leads people to think that "their" fatigue finally has an answer, if not a remedy.

Dr. Kirk suggests that when such announcements are made, people should look carefully at the characteristics of the patients studied. A close reading, he says, nearly always shows that patients were carefully selected, with any patient showing psychiatric or depressive symptoms ruled out. "The bad message that gets communicated when small groups of people may have a particular viral condition is that everybody decides that everyone has it."

FATIGUE USED TO MONGER OTHER DISEASES

The pharmaceutical industry cannot take the blame for chronic fatigue syndrome: if it's considered to be due to a virus, there's no drug that treats viruses very well. But the drug industry, as well as groups mongering other diseases, can use the ubiquitous symptom of fatigue as if it is a fairly specific sign of the disease they are trying to sell you. Consider, for example, a 1990 advertisement from Sigma-Tau pharmaceuticals that features a rag doll slumped by a windowpane on which condensed water conveys a sense of chill. "The Silent Energy Crisis," it trumpets. "The lethargic, hypotonic child. The fretful infant who doesn't eat. No specific evidence of disease . . . yet something clearly is wrong."

The ad goes on to say that pediatricians are now identifying a cause of these and other similarly perplexing symptoms, an inability to metabolize fatty acids that may be due to a deficiency of a substance in the body known as carnitine. One cause of this problem is primary systemic carnitine deficiency. The ad goes on to list a number of conditions that may be associated with carnitine deficiency (even though it has already identified the condition as being associated with no specific evidence of disease). "Because oral carnitine therapy has been proven effective in primary systemic carnitine deficiency in children and because it has little or no toxicity, CARNITOR (levocarnitine) should be considered in all *suspected* [italics added] cases of this syndrome." The ad goes on to say that Carnitor is so safe that there are no contraindications.

The ad is a clear invitation to try the drug for anything and everything; if there are few side effects, why not?

In reality, says Dr. Gunnar B. Stickler, professor emeritus of pediatrics at the Mayo Clinic in Rochester, Minnesota, carnitine deficiency is very rare. In addition, carnitine will normally be provided in the diet, and in any case its deficiency cannot be diagnosed without a thorough investigation.

Nearly all disease-mongering messages include fatigue as a symptom of the disease in question, and it usually is. The posters in the subway touting fatigue as a symptom of lupus erythematosus, the milk cartons saying it could be a sign of diabetes, and the press release telling me it could be the sign of liver disease are technically correct. But it's probably not going to help depressed people to think that they may have a chronic and possibly fatal disease in addition to their depression. It may also lead them astray as to the best way to seek treatment, since depression is treatable with either drugs or cognitive-behavior therapy, and some of the other diseases of which fatigue is a sign are not.

Dr. Kirk advises patients who suffer fatigue to sit down with a doctor who knows them and who may perform a simple exam. While the doctor may turn up some easily treatable explanation, like anemia or hypothyroidism, he or she probably won't, and the fatigue will remain unexplained. The best thing to do then, says Dr. Kirk, is "to get on with your life."

As Dr. Richard D. Huhn wrote in a letter to the *Annals of Internal Medicine*: "In the case of chronic fatigue syndromes (as with other mysterious maladies) the best course is for physician and patient to be able to say 'I don't know.' There is not always an explanation and there is not always a solution: The patient must be made to understand this and then he or she must accept the situation as best as possible and, perhaps, laugh at it."

Chapter 9

Allergy to Life and Everything Else

Knock: 'To fall ill,' is an old notion that doesn't hold up in the face of the facts of modern science. Health is just a word, which it would not be inconvenient to scratch from our vocabulary. In my opinion, I only know people more or less affected by diseases more or less numerous that progress more or less rapidly.
—Jules Romains, *Knock*

Don Jewitt, M.D., a professor of orthopedic surgery at the University of California at San Francisco, was convinced he was on to something. He suffered from multiple symptoms that seemed to be allergic, and while treatment from an orthodox allergist had helped initially, after a while his symptoms were back at full force. He sought out a specialist in clinical ecology, a discipline that broadens the concept of allergy to include many substances such as petrochemicals for which the tests of orthodox allergists do not detect the classic immune responses. The treatment, which consisted in part of excluding certain substances from the diet and from the environment, seemed to be helping him. Dr. Jewett was also treating patients with the approach, and it seemed to be working for them as well.

Because of his successes, Dr. Jewitt decided that he would show the world that the treatments used by clinical ecologists indeed worked and perhaps even how they worked. "I thought I could show that it worked, and if it did, I would explain all the things that modern medicine couldn't. I even thought I might win the Nobel prize."

One of the major procedures used in clinical ecology is known as the symptom provocation test. In this test, various substances are injected under the skin. If the patient then experiences symptoms such as nasal stuffiness, dry mouth, nausea, fatigue, headache, and feelings of disorientation or depression, the clinical ecologist diagnoses an allergy to the particular substance. Clinical ecologists sometimes then give a different dilution (sometimes more, sometimes less concentrated) to neutralize the symptoms.

A major criticism of this technique is that patients obviously know that they are getting a substance of some sort injected under their skin, and in medicine there is not only a placebo effect, in which patients can be healed by an inert substance, but also a negative placebo effect, where inert substances cause noxious symptoms. It's the same power of suggestion that convinces medical students to develop symptoms of the diseases they are studying. Dr. Jewett devised a double-blind test of the method, where neither patients nor their doctors would know whether they were getting the active substance or the inert substance, and whether it was intended to provoke the symptoms or to neutralize them.

Before performing the experiments, Dr. Jewett made sure to show the protocol to both clinical ecologists and orthodox scientists to make certain it was airtight. Clinical ecologists liked the study design because it duplicated the way they ordinarily performed the tests; in addition, the patients selected were known to be ones who ordinarily responded well to the tests. Orthodox scientists liked it, too, because it was double-blinded.

When he actually performed the study, much to Dr. Jewitt's surprise, it made no difference whether patients got the active substance or the placebo. While patients judged 27 percent of the injections of active substance to be active substance, they judged 24 percent of the inert injections to be active, too. The neutralizing doses given by some of the physicians worked just as well if they were placebo as if they were the supposedly active substance.

Dr. Jewitt had to admit that both the symptoms provoked and

their neutralization were due not to allergies to specific substances, but to a very nonspecific placebo effect stemming from
the fact that both patients and doctors believed in the method.
Indeed, Dr. Jewitt now believes that much of so-called modern
medicine works via the placebo effect and that a great many of
the symptoms people suffer today are nonspecific responses to
stress rather than specific allergies to specific substances. His
own so-called allergic symptoms, he says, were particularly acute
when he was going through a divorce and greatly improved when
he remarried. When he thought about the patients he had treated
with the methods of clinical ecology, he says, he now realizes
that many of them showed the classic helplessness and hope-
lessness displayed by depressed patients, and he believes this
probably accounted for many of their symptoms. "The treatment
worked when I was enthusiastic, and didn't when I lost my
enthusiasm."

When Dr. Jewett presented his report to the association of
clinical ecologists six years ago, they became very defensive,
accusing him of being an enemy. "The people who complained
the most were the ones making the most money," he says. But
he doesn't think that most clinical ecologists are in the field only
to exploit their patients. "They're like everyone else," he says.
"They remember the times they've won, and forget the times
they lost." In addition, he says, there's a considerable process of
self-selection between doctor and patient. "If you tell a patient
that their symptoms are due to the food they eat and they look
skeptical, they probably won't come back. But if their face lights
up, and they say 'Oh, really?' then the treatment will probably
work because it coincides with their belief system."

But while the clinical ecologists may mean well, with their
battery of nonobjective tests they have expanded the concept of
allergy in true mongering fashion to include more people, allergic
to more substances. Sometimes this includes "all chemicals" or
all substances of low molecular weight. Some patients make
major changes in their life-style to avoid the chemicals in question,
and some even jeopardize their life.

Consider a woman seen by John C. Selner, M.D., and Herman
Staudenmayer, Ph.D., of the Allergy Respiratory Institute of
Colorado in Denver. This woman had had metastatic cancer of

the bowel when she was in her late thirties, and about nine years later developed a recurrence of cancer. She also had hay fever, and she went to a well-known California ecologist to investigate it. During the tests, she talked to another patient who told of suddenly being unable to tolerate a number of chemicals and foods, explaining to the woman that this was a common experience for ecologically-ill patients. This belief was subsequently reinforced by the physician.

Ten days later the woman began experiencing multiple chemical intolerances to substances such as natural gas, formaldehyde, phenols, and petrochemicals and to many foods. While the woman requested admission to the unit in Denver, the Denver doctors referred her to a doctor in her area, who discovered progression of her cancer and referred her to an oncologist. The oncologist in turn encouraged Drs. Selner and Staudenmayer to admit the woman, because, thinking she was allergic to many foods, she was refusing to eat and had lost one-third of her body weight; her oncologist felt she would starve to death before her cancer would kill her.

She was admitted, and Drs. Selner and Staudenmayer found that rather than having multiple allergies, she was unable to cope with the reality of dying with unfulfilled life expectations. She was placed on a sound diet and given intense psychotherapy. "At six months follow-up, she had returned to her usual endeavors, was again enjoying the symphony and gourmet dining, and had gained an additional 15 pounds. Our last report was received from the beach at Maui."

Clinical ecologists are so successful, Drs. Selner and Staudemayer explained, because people have learned to expect an explanation for all their symptoms and ills. "The failure to produce answers, in spite of incredible advances on the part of medical science and major monetary commitments by both industry and government, has tended to spawn suspicion in the minds of the public," they wrote in *Psychobiological Aspects of Allergic Disorders*. "The ecologists offer a philosophy of certainty. They are certain of cause and course of virtually all presenting disease states. Often they reassure patients on the basis of an initial phone contact that their diagnosis is obviously ecologic disease."

ALLERGY TO CANDIDA ALBICANS

A variant of the environmental allergy syndrome is the allergy to the fungal infections known as *Candida albicans*. Here, though, the focus is on natural, rather than artificial substances. Many women have *Candida albicans* in their vaginas, which sometimes flare up, causing itching and burning, discharge, and odor. In some cases the symptoms are so slight that women aren't bothered very much and don't need to seek treatment; in other cases doctors will prescribe an antifungal agent. But while there's no question that *Candida albicans* can cause vaginal symptoms, and sometimes symptoms in the gastrointestinal tract, recently some doctors have claimed that a condition they call chronic candidiasis causes everything from premenstrual syndrome to depression, proposing a treatment that ranges from a diet that eliminates sugar and yeast products (including bread) to intensive treatment with antifungal products. Some of these doctors reportedly diagnose everyone with the same affliction—everyone, that is, who can pay the nearly $900 some of them charge for a first visit.

To try to gain credibility for the disease of chronic candidiasis, one of its foremost proponents, C. Orian Truss, M.D., of the Critical Illness Research Foundation in Birmingham, Alabama, approached a professor of infectious disease at the University of Alabama, Dr. William E. Dismukes. Dr. Truss asked Dr. Dismukes to perform a study that would show once and for all whether the treatment, which consisted of eliminating many foods from the diet as well as therapy with the antifungal agent nystatin, worked. Dr. Dismukes agreed, and he and his colleagues devised a study design that they showed to Dr. Truss, letting Dr. Truss identify patients presumed to have the syndrome, 42 premenopausal women, for the study. In order to simplify the results, Dr. Dismukes and his colleages did not test the diet, but instead divided the women into four groups, giving one group oral nystatin, another group a placebo to take orally, a third group vaginal nystatin, and a fourth group a vaginal placebo. While the nystatin proved much more effective in clearing up the local systems of vaginal infections, the placebos proved just as good as the nystatin when it came to improving the mood and PMS supposedly caused by the chronic candidiasis, causing Dr. Dismukes and his colleagues to conclude that any effect of the nystatin on mood and PMS must be a placebo one.

Dr. Dismukes doesn't believe that most of the doctors promoting chronic candidiasis as a disease are insincere, since he believes, like Dr. Jewett, that a lot of medicine has to do with environments and situations. Nor does he believe that those who insist they suffer from chronic candidiasis are doing themselves any physical harm by the treatment, although they spend lots of money both to take the drug and to avoid contact with all the things that supposedly cause their symptoms. "There are a lot of yeasts, molds, and fungi in the world, and you can't avoid them," he explains. He bases his belief that nystatin is harmless on the fact that his study showed that nystatin is not absorbed into the body from the gut. While this means it is unlikely to have much effect on symptoms elsewhere in the body, it also means it is unlikely to be highly toxic.

CHILDHOOD ALLERGIES

Believing that your own symptoms are due to multiple allergies can be expensive, and occasionally, as we saw in the case of the woman with cancer, life draining and even life threatening. But some people insist that they feel better if they avoid the offending substances, and they therefore probably should: After all, whose life is it, anyway?

But putting innocent children on such diets when the evidence for their necessity is weak and when children themselves probably would not choose to forego many of the substances being restricted is another matter.

Gunnar B. Stickler, M.D., retired chairman of pediatrics at the Mayo Clinic, says he himself is allergic to the millions of food allergies, the uncounted cases of milk allergy, the ecologists, and the sublingualists (referring to ecologists who test their patients by putting the offending substances under the tongue). He believes that for every 100 children diagnosed with food allergy, only one child truly has one.

While Dr. Stickler has a special quarrel with the methods of clinical ecologists, orthodox allergists are not much better, he says, since they, too, often fail to diagnose allergies with the rigors of a double-blind test; instead they simply take a history and then give a simple challenge test, which the parents and children know is the food to which they are supposed to be allergic.

> My special allergy flared again the other day when I saw a fine-looking 4-year-old boy who was in the 25th percentile for height and weight after almost a year of Isomil, rice bread, "low-acid orange juice," and peanut butter prescribed because he had too many colds, earaches, and itches and had become oppositional. In addition, he had received sublingual desensitization. My treatment was simple: he was placed on a general diet—without explosive consequences; and I acquired a new friend who can now eat doughnuts and bread again, and many other foods he has missed.
>
> Perhaps the time may come when a physician will be accused of child abuse when performing numerous skin tests, assigning a tightly restricted menu, and continuing a steady diet of desensitizations instead of normal food."

Occasionally it's the parents who seem to be abusing their children by keeping them on a restrictive diet justified by "allergies." Researchers in England recruited parents who had eliminated the yellow dye tartrazine from their children's diet after reading articles in the press that it caused disorders such as hyperactivity. The parents were all convinced that their children became hyperactive after eating or drinking something that contained tartrazine—until the researchers had them observe their child's behavior and they were not able to tell whether their child had drunk orange juice containing tartrazine or just orange juice.

Most of the parents found the study convincing enough to put their children back on a normal diet. But the parents of three patients balked. "The parents of one patient, who was only on three foods at the time of admission, were unable to accept that the child was not food intolerant, and when new items of food were added to the diet they insisted that as a result the child had loose stools, skin rashes, and an adverse behavioral change, although none of these events were detectable to the nursing or medical staff. This child remained on a very restricted diet against our wishes."

But the good news from the English study was that the parents of the other 21 children responded to the demonstration and returned their children to a normal diet. These parents had only been trying to do the best for their children, responding in what seemed a logical manner to the information they were getting. Diseases can be easily mongered, but they can also be de-mongered when physicians are willing to take the time to do so.

Chapter 10

Creating Cardiac Cripples I

"Silent" Myocardial Ischemia: Should You Take A Stress Test?

I was driving along a sun-dappled road. The full panoply of nature's new greens exploded before me. From the radio came one of Mozart's gifts to the spirit. It was the kind of day that makes you count your blessings.

Suddenly, there was a subliminal tampering with my psyche: the music changed. Half a dozen bopping sounds warned me that danger lurked, and a man's moonsilver voice—signifying that what he was saying was for my own good—told me that, at any moment, my heart might—more bopping—STOP! But, he says, I can be saved, thanks to the doctors at a certain hospital who know how to wield the latest laser technology on my clogged arteries. . . .

. . . I know that in order to reap the benefits of new forms of technology we must first know about them. But what comes across in these radio spots is something besides education. An underlying voice says: 'The medical buck is getting harder to come by. Spend it with us.'
—Irene Fischl, *New England Journal of Medicine*, 1989.

Thomas Graboys, M.D., of Lown Cardiovascular Laboratories at the Harvard School of Public Health, tells the story of a healthy and entirely asymptomatic 45-year-old man who reluctantly agreed to undergo a "heart screening" at the local YMCA. When the electrocardiogram was found to be abnormal, the doctor ordered, in succession, ambulatory electrocardiographic monitoring, an exercise thallium imaging of the heart, coronary angiography (an X ray of the coronary artery, a procedure that carries with it a slight, but real, chance of dying), and an angioplasty (a procedure that will temporarily clear the arteries but in at least 40 percent of cases won't keep them clear). Four hours after the angioplasty, the man for the first time experienced severe substernal chest pressure. Six months later, he died suddenly.

Many doctors and patients may answer that the man would have certainly died in any case, and perhaps they are right. But the poor record of angioplasty, due perhaps to the fact that it destroys tissues in the lining of blood vessels that produce important regulatory chemicals, makes the opposite conclusion equally plausible. Medical science cannot answer for certain what would have happened to this man if he had not had the stress test that led to all the other procedures. Indeed, it does not yet have even the statistical answers: What would happen to 100 apparently healthy men who had a stress test, and what would happen to 100 healthy men who didn't?

Such a vacuum of information is fertile soil for disease mongering.

When they become anxious, many people develop chest pains, which make them ready targets for expensive tests and potentially dangerous procedures. But "silent" myocardial ischemia, alias "silent" heart disease, is an even better concept for modern Dr. Knocks since you don't even have to have symptoms for it. As one doctor pointed out in an article by Sandra Blakeslee in the *New York Times*, there are 20 to 40 million middle-aged Americans and while most are healthy, they should not consider themselves immune to coronary artery disease.

It's true that you can feel perfectly well right now, yet drop dead tomorrow, or even today. But mongers play with this truth in two ways. One is to exaggerate the probability that this will happen. The other is to imply that medical science necessarily has a solution.

A good many people stand to profit from convincing the healthy that they should start the process that may eventually label them as diseased: cardiologists, the number of whom more than doubled between 1970 and 1987; manufacturers of the equipment used for stress tests and for angioplasty; and cardiologists in training, who need a group of relatively healthy patients on whom to practice their skills. Dr. Graboys tells of one cardiologist who suggested that his colleagues who were learning how to perform angioplasty should select patients with simple single-vessel disease, normal ventricular function, and an age of less than 70 years. "This is precisely the profile of an individual with coronary disease who is likely to exhibit an excellent outcome when treated medically—i.e., the least likely candidate for angioplasty," Dr. Graboys wrote in the *Journal of the American Medical Association*. "In the search for patients, the population of asymptomatic individuals with silent ischemia is becoming a suitable pool from which to draw."

Drug companies advertise: "In myocardial ischemia, treat the patient when he feels the pain and when he doesn't." Jane Brody, in her personal health column in the *New York Times*, tells us about silent heart disease, a painless condition that poses great peril for millions of Americans. Not until we are well into the column do we learn that only people who have known risk factors for heart disease ought to be tested, and even further down in the column that even when silent myocardial ischemia is diagnosed, nobody really knows whether it should be treated.

"At present there are no data on which to base a management approach for the true silent ischemic," says Dr. Graboys. Yet the climate of publicity created by cardiologists and medical writers makes it seem as if everyone should have, at the very least, a stress test. In 1988 the mongering fire was fueled even further when an arbitration panel composed of lawyers in Los Angeles County ruled in favor of a family's $500,000 malpractice suit against a primary care physician who neglected to test for coronary artery disease in a 40-year-old man, who a few days after his physical examination died suddenly while jogging—even though a stress test was unlikely to predict this man's death.

All of these pressures make it difficult for the non mongering physician who recognizes that the stress test to identify silent myocardial ischemia, particularly in individuals who are at low risk of heart disease, may lead to more problems than it solves. As Dr. Graboys wrote in the *Journal of the American Medical*

Association: "Conservative management is viewed frequently as antiquated and suboptimal, particularly when the menu of interventions is varied and appealing"—and expensive.

"NOISY" ISCHEMIA

To understand the controversy over silent myocardial ischemia, it is first necessary to understand a little bit about myocardial ischemia that is not silent. When the arteries that supply the heart with blood are in some way blocked, the heart suffers and often lets the person know by causing pain. If the heart is getting sufficient oxygen to live, the pain takes the form of angina pectoris. If the heart is getting so little oxygen that it is being damaged, a heart attack, or myocardial infarction, is taking place, often resulting in crushing chest pains.

Treatment of angina has two purposes: to make the patient feel better and to try to reduce the chances that the heart will be damaged. Success in the first case can be assessed only by the patient. Success in the second can be assessed only by clinical trials that show that people who are treated are less likely to die or to have more progressive disease.

It is perfectly justified and desirable to make people aware that chest pains can be serious so that they can seek help immediately and perhaps save their lives. But one problem that hasn't been adequately addressed is that in a fairly significant proportion of people who have chest pains, the pains are not due to heart problems at all; they are due to anxiety or to problems originating in the stomach, esophagus, or skeletal muscles. One estimate is that the average patient complaining of chest pain to a practitioner is 15 to 100 times more likely to be anxious than to have heart disease. Chest pains and palpitations are among the top five symptoms unexplained by any physical cause, and even after extensive testing of chest pains severe enough that the doctor believed further testing necessary, no organic reason can be found in about 30 percent of patients. For these people, the tests will be dangerous without any concomitant benefits. In 1984, for example, approximately 540,000 heart catheterizations, known as angiographies, were performed, of which 10 to 45 percent showed the person had a normal coronary artery. The death rate from angiography is about 0.1 percent, meaning that even if the lower figure is the correct one, 54 people who had no heart disease died from their angiography.

Ironically, many of those who live through the test and are found to have no evidence of heart disease continue to believe that they do. According to one study, reported in the *American Journal of Cardiology*, two-thirds of patients who were found to have normal coronary arteries continued to believe they had heart disease, with many doctors continuing to treat them as heart patients and to prescribe cardiac medications. A total of 86 percent said they continued to have chest pain at least once a week, 71 percent said their pain was unchanged or worse, and 63 percent were still being treated for their chest pain. Another researcher found that some patients with normal tests continued to believe that they had heart disease, thus limiting their activities and fearing exertion. In this study, after a normal catheterization, 32 percent described themselves as limited in physical activity, 45 percent considered exertion dangerous, and 30 percent received cardiac drugs. While 47 percent of the sample were told their symptoms were due to stress only 4 percent were told to see a professional. In one group, 55 percent believed they had experienced a heart attack, despite the fact that only 2 percent had been so told in the past.

To add to the difficulties, anxiety can induce changes in the so-called objective measures of heart disease. Anxious people may hyperventilate, for example, which can produce a blip on the electrocardiogram known as a T-wave change, which doctors not adequately trained in interpretation may read as a manifestation of heart disease.

While we can't really fault public information campaigns that let people know that chest pains may be serious, or physicians who perform a certain number of tests on people whose chest pains are due to anxiety, clearly there's a problem here. Perhaps those in charge of informing the public need to emphasize that while it's important to have chest pains checked out, they aren't necessarily serious. People whose chest pains don't seem to be due to heart disease probably need a lot more reassurance than they're currently getting.

SILENT ISCHEMIA

The discovery that many patients have changes on their exercise electrocardiogram (stress test) that are similar to those seen in patients with angina and that such changes do predict an increased risk of heart disease led to the concept of "silent" heart disease. The pharmaceutical firms that made drugs used to treat angina were quick to conclude that if the pain of angina should be treated with their drugs, so should the painless changes similar to those seen with angina. This conclusion was not without its logic. But of the two reasons to treat "noisy" ischemia—to reduce pain and to prevent long-term deterioration—only one is present in silent ischemia since there is no pain. As an article by Drs. Prakash C. Deedwania and Enrique V. Carbajal in the *Archives of Internal Medicine* points out, conventional anti-angina therapy does not eliminate the silent episodes; in addition, "whether treatment of silent ischemia can alter the associated adverse prognosis is not known."

According to Harold Sox, M.D., chairman of medicine at Dartmouth-Hitchcock Medical Center in Lebanon, New Hampshire, physicians know very little about coronary artery disease in people with no symptoms. "We don't know their frequency of severe disease, and we have no idea whether bypass surgery or angioplasty alters their long-term prognosis."

Since the results of treating silent heart disease with antianginal drugs, bypass surgery, or angioplasty are unknown, does it really help to make the diagnosis? According to Dr. David Pryor, an associate professor of medicine at Duke University in Durham, North Carolina, people with no symptoms to relieve and usually at low risk for the short term, "have little to gain from the diagnosis except motivation for reducing risk factors."

IS A STRESS TEST WORTH THE STRESS?

A stress test in itself, which consists of walking on a treadmill while your electrocardiogram is monitored, is probably pretty low risk, although the author of the French *Asterix* books died during one (the doctors responded that he certainly would have died very soon anyway, a response that might—or might not—

have been correct). But the stress test diagnoses silent ischemia—and as we have just seen, there's no agreement as to what to do about it.

While the stress test itself is probably low risk, it is also not very sensitive or specific, and many doctors don't know how to interpret it. According to Dr. Myrvin Ellestad, director of research at the Memorial Heart Institute in Long Beach, California, "Perhaps 10 percent of the doctors who do exercise tests are fully informed about the test's nuances. There are all sorts of degrees of abnormality, and the real problem is not in doing it, but in knowing what to do when it's done."

This means that while it is sometimes accurate, it labels as healthy many people who do have heart disease and labels as sick many people who don't. The first group may be falsely reassured (although since reassurance may be at a premium in the world, perhaps it's not so bad to be reassured if you can't do anything about the condition) and the second group started on a round of follow-up tests that may prove more dangerous than their initial risk. "The majority of persons destined to die suddenly will not have a positive exercise test," according to Dr. Stephen Epstein, chief of cardiology at the National Institutes of Health in Bethesda, Maryland. Screening people who have no symptoms and have not had a previous heart attack "in the hope of preventing sudden coronary death will be largely futile."

Journalist Dan Levin, writing in *Sports Illustrated*, recalled his own stress test:

> After 10 minutes on the treadmill, the stress test and EKG [electrocardiogram] nearly complete and indicating nothing untoward, the doctor injected the thallium intravenously, and that set in motion a chain of events that would last seven weeks. In that stretch I would have five more tests, including two that I would fail and another that has killed more than a few people. I would have personal consultations with four cardiologists, including one who would say that I very likely had coronary artery disease, and two more who would say that I almost certainly did not. And as the weeks passed, I would grow more and more reclusive and despairing. I would be unable to work, fearful that each halting step might be my last. Finally, after running up a medical bill of $8,983 ($8,023 of it going for the tests, and most of it covered by various medical plans), I would receive assurance that my

coronary arteries were normal, that the pains had almost certainly been of musculoskeletal origin.

In general, the more risk factors you have for heart disease, the more valuable a stress test will be, since if you remember Baye's rule from chapter 3, the lower your risk, the more likely a positive test will be falsely positive. But even when physicians restrict exercise tests to people with a certain number of risk factors, rather than giving it willy-nilly to everyone, it's still pretty arbitrary. According to Mitchell L. Zoler, writing in *Medical World News*, a task force of the American College of Cardiology and the American Heart Association couldn't identify a single circumstance "for which there is general agreement that exercise testing is justified." One study found that of 20 asymptomatic people who have an abnormal ST response on an exercise electrocardiogram (EKG), only one will have a "hard" cardiac event such as a heart attack in the next five to eight years after the test. "This means that 19 out of 20 must deal with the psychological, social, and financial problems created by a false-positive test," according to Dr. Victor Froelicher, professor at Palo Alto Veterans Affairs Medical Center. If people who have the abnormal ST response go on to angiography and some of them have bypass surgery or angioplasty, there's a 40-percent chance that the bypass will occlude within five to eight years and they'll have to have another.

One common negative effect of a false-positive test is that people may be afraid to exercise, when exercise may be the best thing they could do for their hearts. "Too much testing is unwise," wrote Bernard Gutin, Ph.D., then professor of applied physiology and education at Columbia University's Teachers College. "A remarkably large number of tests for ischemic heart disease in young and middle-aged women have been falsely positive." This has misled many women into becoming "cardiac cripples" who fear to exercise.

If the lack of exercise does not increase the risk of a heart attack, the anxiety created by a false-positive test may. While the role of emotions in heart disease remains to be understood, at least one study found that among people who have already had one heart attack, certain emotional states were accurate predictors of second heart attacks. In men, hostility and anger were found to be most important, while in women, anxiety, fearfulness, and phobias were more powerful predictors. The same researchers suspected that depression and low self-esteem were involved in both instances.

Such considerations were at play when the British Civil Aviation Authority decided not to have its airline pilots routinely undergo stress testing. Wrote G. Bennett, the chief medical officer, in a letter to the *British Medical Journal*: "There has not been a major airline accident from physical incapacitation of a pilot in more than 15 years and 200 million flying hours." This has occurred, he explained, because backup procedures have been developed to take over when a pilot has been incapacitated—something that will occasionally occur no matter what medical tests the pilots have undergone.

Dr. Bennett went on to point out that 76 percent of all accidents—and 53 percent of fatal accidents—are due to human error. "We clearly need pilots who are free of worry even more than we need those free of coronary artery disease." Routine exercise electrocardiography, he pointed out, would just contribute to their worries.

So if you are healthy and don't have symptoms, a stress test probably offers you very little except additional stress in your life. If you *are* having symptoms, you may not need a stress test, since you will probably move on to other tests. "It's the patient with atypical symptoms—funny chest pains—for whom exercise testing adds the most information," says Dr. Ellestad. Dr. Thomas Pickering, of New York Hospital, says that a stress test *can* help patients who have already had heart attacks avoid the more dangerous angiography: "If I have a patient who has had an MI, I feel more secure about not ordering coronary angiography if I know that he or she can 'pass' an exercise test before leaving the hospital."

Despite the limited value of stress tests, they continue to increase, with Medicare records showing a 22 percent increase in testing from 1986 to 1988.

"SILENT" LEG PAIN

The arteries that control the blood supply to the arms and legs can also become clogged. If they become completely occluded, the tissues of the limb will die, and the limb will have to be amputated. If they become partly occluded, they may cause the pain known as intermittent claudication, a situation comparable in cause to the pain of angina, which can often be treated by exercise and by stopping smoking. Just as there is "silent" ischemia in the heart, there can be partial occlusion of the arteries carrying blood to the legs that does not result in any pain.

Traditionally, peripheral vascular disease has been treated conservatively, and exercise and stopping smoking have worked for most people. Jay Coffman, M.D., of Boston University Medical Center pointed out in an editorial in the *New England Journal of Medicine* that in several studies, about 75 percent of patients with intermittent claudication had stable symptoms or even improved over a period of four to nine years without intervention. "Several well-controlled studies have shown that exercise regimens increase the distance patients with intermittent claudication are able to walk. After a few months of walking for 30 to 60 minutes every day or every other day, patients' maximal walking distance may increase remarkably. Some have increased the distance they can walk from 1 city block to 10 blocks without leg pain."

Traditionally, if these conservative measures weren't sufficient, vascular surgeons would operate to improve the circulation. Since surgery was risky, they were inclined to intervene only when the patient's disease threatened loss of a limb. More recently, interventional radiologists, a relatively new type of specialist have started treating peripheral vascular disease, since they are able to treat the disease at the same time they diagnose it with radiology techniques. Interventional radiologists may be inclined to treat patients with less serious disease, since the risks of unclogging the blood vessels are less than of replacing the vessels surgically. But disease mongering is kept low in this instance because most people don't usually go to a radiologist directly but are usually referred by someone else, which tends to put a brake on unnecessary procedures. There are only about 2,000 interventional radiologists in the country, who typically have extensive training in peripheral procedures.

What some people find troubling is that cardiologists, the number of whom increased from 3,882 in 1970 to 9,925 in 1987, are also becoming interested in peripheral vascular surgery, meaning that vascular surgeons, interventional radiologists, and cardiologists have begun to fight over the available patients in what has been called the vascular wars. Perhaps this is why, in Maryland, the number of angioplasty procedures performed for peripheral vascular disease of the lower extremities increased several-fold in the decade between 1979 and 1989, and interestingly, the large number of these procedures lowered neither the incidence of the more major bypass operations, which doubled during the same time period, nor the rate of amputation of the limbs, which remained the same. Dr. Coffman speculated that the complications of angioplasty procedures might themselves have led to amputations in a few cases.

The entry of cardiologists into the field is troubling for several reasons, according to the interventional radiologists and the vascular surgeons: (1) there are lots of cardiologists trying to find adequate patient loads; (2) patients generally go directly to cardiologists, who have a financial interest in recommending procedures that they can perform themselves; (3) most cardiologists by their own admission have typically not studied much about the peripheral circulation in their residency training programs; and (4) cardiologists—after a two-day training course—may want to "practice" on the legs before they attempt catheterizing the heart. "The legs have become a training ground for cardiologists, and patients are being subjected not only to unproved technology but to procedures performed by those with little expertise or appropriate previous experience," wrote D. Eugene Strandness, Jr., M.D., of the University of Washington School of Medicine, in the journal *Radiology.*

Responsible cardiologists recognize that if their specialty is to take on these procedures, they at least should start getting significant training in them. But, as reported in the *Journal of the American College of Cardiology,* "it is recognized that hospitals are currently under intense pressure to grant privileges to cardiologists who have not had adequate training so as to protect the hospitals' referral base."

Eric Martin, M.D., an interventional radiologist at Columbia-Presbyterian Medical Center in New York, explains that sometimes when physicians perform a coronary angiogram of the coronary artery, they'll look at the peripheral blood vessels, whether or not the patient has complained of pain. "It has been known for them to say 'you have a stenosis and I should dilate it.' But nobody really knows how to manage these 'silent' stenoses, and if the patient doesn't complain, it's not significant to them."

Adding to the pressure to look for trivial disease are the companies that market ultrasound systems, such as the one mentioned in chapter 4 that pointed out to doctors just how much they could add to their income by the tests alone.

But while treating trivial disease may be easy, it's not totally risk free, says Ernest Ring, M.D., professor of radiology at the University of California at San Francisco, who testifies in court as an expert five or six times a year when someone has botched the procedure. "If the iliac artery is ruptured, the patient usually dies."

For a while, the gimmick used to recruit patients was the laser, since patients tend to believe that lasers are magic. But there is no evidence that lasers are any better than conventional tools for performing these procedures, and doctors who advertised that they used lasers often used them simply as a heat source or as a mechanical device for pushing through the occlusion without even turning on the laser. Nevertheless, a variety of "institutes" and "centers" for laser therapy sprang up throughout the United States to attract patients with peripheral vascular disease, often directed by physicians with minimal previous experience or training in this field. When the FDA approved certain lasers, this, too, was used as a marketing tool, although as we saw in chapter 3 the FDA approval of a device does not necessarily mean that its use benefits the patient.

As Christopher K. Zarins, M.D., wrote in the *Journal of the American Medical Association*: "Aggressive marketing practices and two-day teaching programs to demonstrate ease of use and profitability have spurred enormous interest. As a result, many lesions that never have required treatment are being aggressively sought out and treated."

As a consequence, he wrote, patients whose symptoms are not that troublesome—and in the past were treated by trying to get them to stop smoking and to start walking—are now undergoing invasive procedures. Besides the fact that no one knows what will happen to these patients in the long term, "no evidence exists to support the rationale that the early treatment of asymptomatic superficial femoral lesions, which are technically easy to treat and economically rewarding, is of benefit to the patient."

So what do you do? Certainly, avoid those centers that advertise laser surgery, or indeed advertise at all. If you're worried about heart disease, either because you have chest pains or because you're just worried, try to find a family practitioner, internist, or noninterventional cardiologist (one who doesn't perform procedures much more complicated than an electrocardiogram) who doesn't have a financial interest in performing any of the procedures and who doesn't own stock in the centers to which he or she refers you for testing. Make it clear that you want to know what conditions any tests recommended test for, whether these conditions are treatable, and whether there is in fact any point in taking the test. Life is fraught, as a friend of mine likes to say, but you should determine whether in your particular case embarking on a series of tests may be more fraught than doing nothing at all. If all you stand to gain from the procedures is motivation to exercise, to give up smoking, and to watch your diet a little more, do you really need the tests to tell you this?

Chapter 11

Creating Cardiac Cripples II

Murmurs, Mitral Valve Prolapse, and Arrhythmias

My grandmother worried her whole life about her heart murmur, and died at the age of 90.
—Susan Walton, Hers column, *New York Times*, June 25, 1987.

Have you your stethoscope? Might I ask you—would you have the kindness? I have grave doubts as to my mitral valve, if you would be so good. The aortic I may rely upon, but I would value your opinion upon the mitral. I listened to his heart, as requested, but was unable to find anything amiss, save, indeed, that he was in an ecstasy of fear.
—Thaddeus Sholto and John H. Watson, M.D., from the collected works of Sherlock Holmes.

When a 14-year-old New Jersey boy died of a heart attack during soccer practice in 1985, a member of the pathology department at Rancocas Valley Hospital, where the boy was taken, was quoted in the *New York Times* as saying, "He probably had a murmur since birth." The school's athletic director, Richard G.

Ballard, was then quoted as saying that any student with a detected heart murmur is barred from sports competition.

Their words must have shot fear into the hearts of many parents, since nearly all children have heart murmurs at one time or another. The problem here is that "heart murmur" is neither a diagnosis nor a disease, but simply a type of sound a doctor hears when he or she puts the stethoscope to someone's chest. In a few instances a murmur may signify serious heart disease, but in most cases it doesn't mean very much. Dan McNamara, M.D., a pediatric cardiologist at Texas Children's Hospital in Houston, explains children have thin chest walls through which the heart is easily heard. "If the child is exercised, or has a fever, and the room is quiet, you might hear a murmur in any child," he says. "Once physicians start looking for innocent murmurs, one or more such murmurs can be heard in practically all children, and certainly in half of them." Athletes are particularly prone to murmurs, with 30 to 50 percent of athletes showing murmurs because of the normal physiological changes that occur in the heart with exercise.

Nobody can claim that heart murmurs and mitral valve prolapse (MVP), a floppiness of the valve controlling blood flow between the atrial and ventricular chambers of the heart, sometimes associated with murmurs, are diseases being mongered by the pharmaceutical industry, since neither is usually treated with drugs. While the diagnostics industry bears some responsibility for the widespread diagnosis of mitral valve prolapse, the same test that diagnoses MVP often dediagnoses "murmurs," or at least proves their innocence, so that here technology comes out even, and in the hands of those who know how to use it, it *can* play a major role in convincing people who thought they were sick that they are well.

Rather, the responsibility for unnecessary worry about heart murmurs and MVP may be a direct result of the physical examination. When large numbers of people come in with nothing particularly wrong with them, the doctor gets tired of writing that in fact this patient is perfectly well. He or she has been trained to listen to the heart; indeed, the stethoscope is the trademark of the physician. Murmurs are common and probably more common during the stress of a medical visit, and so the doctor hears and records them. Gunnar B. Stickler, M.D., professor emeritus of pediatrics at the Mayo Clinic, put it this way: "Where are the times when the record of a physical examination read: 'This 5-year-old girl looks well, she is happy, and there is no abnormal physical finding'?

"Many of the patients seen have a dull or red tympanic membrane [eardrum] or at least some fluid behind the drum. There are 'hypertrophic'[enlarged] tonsils, or the submandibular nodes [lymph nodes below the jawbone] are enlarged. The heart attracts most attention. Since we have a scale of 1 to 6 with which to grade murmurs, there is very often at least a grade 1 systolic murmur mentioned."

THE EMPEROR'S CLOTHES SYNDROME

While hearing a murmur appears to depend more on the conditions of the room than of the heart, it can also be a side effect of what Frank Gross, M.D., defined in the *New England Journal of Medicine* as the Emperor's Clothes Syndrome. According to Dr. Gross, the Emperor's Clothes Syndrome was being seen in almost epidemic form in cardiology and neurology departments. Typically, the syndrome occurs when the chief is making rounds with four residents and three interns. The chief listens to the heart and hears a murmur. Nobody else hears it, but after the senior resident says, "I heard it," the setting is perfect for a mini-epidemic. "Down the line, in rapid succession, members of the group are infected. The diagnosis can easily be made by the pathogenic sign, 'I hear it.'"

The problem is that some doctors still don't seem to understand the significance of hearing a murmur, and still others don't do a very good job of reassuring parents that their child's heart murmur is totally innocent. In 1967, Abraham B. Bergman, M.D., a pediatrician at the University of Washington School of Medicine in Seattle, found that the disability in children falsely perceived as having heart disease was greater than in a comparable group of children who actually had organic lesions of their heart. "A growing child who is restricted from physical activities such as swimming, bicycle riding and other sports is surely as disabled as one with a cast and crutches," he wrote. Another study showed that children falsely labeled with heart disease had impaired intellectual development. Fewer children are probably restricted today, says Martin Alpert, M.D., of the University of South Alabama at Mobile, since the technique of echocardiography makes it easier to distinguish between heart murmurs that signal serious disease and those that are simply innocent or "flow" murmurs. This doesn't mean that every child with a murmur, which means nearly every child, needs an "echo," which can cost $800, but it does mean that if you are told that your child has a heart murmur and should therefore not participate in sports, you should at least consult a cardiologist before you make your child a cardiac cripple.

Dr. McNamara believes that while fewer children are excluded from exercise now, it's not necessarily because pediatricians are better at distinguishing innocent heart murmurs from the others, since he gets a lot of referrals from good, board-certified doctors for heart disease when in fact the child has none. But pediatricians *are* more likely to refer today, and cardiologists can pretty easily distinguish innocent heart murmurs from those that may indicate a serious condition. Parents, however, may be put through a lot of anxiety from the time they're told their child has a murmur until the final tests are performed, and not all cardiologists may give them adequate reassurance that their child's murmur is totally innocent. "It takes a lot of time to explain it," says Dr. McNamara, who explains it by giving parents a sheet of paper to take home with them.

While murmurs due to anxiety are common in children, they are considered rare in adults. I seem to have one, however, and the fact that many doctors do not seem to recognize that the murmur they are hearing is simply a consequence of my anxiety makes me think that perhaps the condition is more common than generally recognized. The problem with having a murmur of any kind is that it is medically "interesting" and tends to be taken more seriously than complaints that seem to the doctor to be more subjective. Joseph D. Wassersug, M.D., notes that "if the patient comes to the office because she's deaf, and we find wax in her ears—but also pick up a mitral systolic click—we get so absorbed in the discovery of a prolapsed mitral valve that we may forget that the prime reason for the visit was ceruminosis" (wax in the ears). In my case, the doctors would listen intently to my heart, tell me I had a murmur, and then say they didn't know what significance it had. One did claim to know the significance, telling me that it was most definitely MVP (without, however, suggesting an echocardiogram, which is the only way to confirm the diagnosis) and that I should take antibiotics whenever I had my teeth cleaned.

I am very resistant to disease mongering and didn't take this too seriously, although the first time I had my teeth cleaned after the diagnosis I felt fragile, and since I am a normally lazy person, I sometimes used the diagnosis as an excuse not to exercise. But no one who heard the murmur ever suggested that it might simply be due to anxiety or even suggested I see a cardiologist. I finally figured out that the murmur was heard only at the consultations where my blood pressure was slightly high and that the two conditions were detected only when I was upset about something.

MITRAL VALVE PROLAPSE

I wrote about my diagnosis of "mitral valve prolapse" in one of my earlier books, *Medicine and Culture*, since at that time I accepted the diagnosis, even though I refused to take antibiotics for it. One night I returned home late to find a message on my answering machine from a young woman who had written a book about how serious a condition MVP was. She obviously thought I would want to know that I had a much more serious condition than I previously thought, and in addition she wanted my suggestions as to who might publish her book. Not too long afterward, a headline over a Jane Brody column in the *New York Times* declared, "Mitral valve prolapse is often called benign. But this common heart disorder can sometimes have life-threatening consequences."

As with many mongered diseases, MVP—otherwise known as a floppy mitral valve—*can* be a serious disease. Richard B. Devereux, M.D., of the New York Hospital-Cornell Medical Center in New York calculates that 4,000 sudden deaths a year may be due to MVP, although this is a small portion—less than 0.1 percent—of the 7 million adults who have the condition. Persons with the condition are at an increased risk of a serious infection of the heart valve known as infectious endocarditis, although most people who develop endocarditis do not have MVP.

But Aubrey Leatham and Wallace Brigden, writing in the *American Heart Journal*, point out that many people thought to have died from MVP usually have something else wrong with their hearts. "In every case where we have been able to find a report on an EKG, it was abnormal," they wrote. "Indeed, we hold the opinion that *isolated* disease of the mitral valve causing mild or moderate reflux [leak] seldom causes symptoms other than those of iatrogenic [doctor-caused] anxiety."

The problem is that there are varying degrees of MVP, ranging from the serious to something that is probably just a slight and entirely benign variant of the normal heart valve. How widespread and how serious the condition is depends on how you define it and particularly what diagnostic methods are used to pick it up. As with most conditions that vary from the serious to the trivial, the more people included in the definition, the less serious the condition becomes.

Consider, for example, defining MVP as the condition of only those people known to have a definite problem resulting from the prolapse of their mitral valve. This would include the 4,000 sudden deaths as well as those who had definite complications such as endocarditis. Defined this way, MVP would be a serious, but relatively rare, disease.

MVP could also be defined as the condition of those individuals who have a certain type of murmur thought to be due to a prolapsed mitral valve, as my own "MVP" was defined. Here the numbers of people with the disease would be large, but very few of them would have a serious complication. (It's impossible to say how many people would be defined as having MVP based on their heart sounds, since people's hearts give different sounds at different times, and doctors' auscultation skills vary widely.)

Since by definition MVP is an anatomical condition, the best way to diagnose it should be by ultrasound, which gives a picture of the anatomy. But when doctors began looking at people using ultrasound (sometimes referred to as echocardiography), they found that huge numbers of seemingly normal people had MVP. Young women and ballet dancers, in particular, are most affected; one study found echocardiographic evidence of MVP in 14 percent of normal young women and 59 percent of female ballet dancers!

But one group of investigators who had found 13 percent of the population had MVP was able to drop it to 0.5 percent when more stringent criteria were employed for making the diagnosis.

"Our reliance on diagnostic tests (particularly echocardiography) to detect mitral-valve prolapse assumes that those tests can distinguish normal from abnormal. But this differentiation is based on arbitrary criteria, since the mobility of the mitral valve is in reality a continuous, not a dichotomous, [either sick or disease] variable," wrote Joshua Wynne, M.D., of Wayne State University, Detroit, in the *New England Journal of Medicine.*

Still another way the diagnosis of MVP can be made is by a group of symptoms known as MVP syndrome. The symptoms are basically those of anxiety, and in fact there appears to be no particular relationship between MVP *syndrome* and the anatomical condition of MVP. The two commonly occur together primarily because both are common. My own experience, where anxiety caused a murmur that was diagnosed as MVP, makes me think that this is probably happening to other people, too.

Dr. Devereux and his colleagues found that only about 7 percent of the people referred to their service with a diagnosis of MVP based on symptoms such as chest pain, difficulty breathing, and panic attacks actually had evidence of a floppy mitral valve as seen by echocardiography.

So when MVP is defined strictly, it can be a serious disease, but when it is defined loosely, it is at most a risk factor, and not a very valid one at that. "Even if these subjects are not truly free of disease, there appears to be no clinical advantage in separating the trivial from the nonexistent," Dr. Wynne wrote in the *New England Journal of Medicine.* Yet the young woman trying to sell her book about MVP was using the most serious consequences: sudden death and endocarditis *and* the definition that included the largest number of people. It was a classic case of disease mongering.

Just why doctors are prone to overdiagnose MVP was illustrated in a candid article by Drs. Timothy E. Quill, Mack Lipkin, Jr., and Philip Greenland in the *Journal of General Internal Medicine.* When the authors were a medical student, a resident, and a junior faculty member at Strong Memorial Hospital in

Rochester, New York, the case of a 35-year-old woman was presented during the hospital's Grand Rounds. The year was 1975, when MVP was first being recognized, described, and treated. The woman had a history of arrhythmias and other heart problems that had necessitated her hospitalization. After an echocardiogram finally showed MVP, the patient underwent surgery, and her symptoms improved remarkably.

The doctors pointed out that this woman—with her dramatic, extreme problems—was typical of the first reported cases of MVP. "It effectively taught that MVP was a disease with a potentially ominous prognosis that physicians should be vigilant to recognize, explore, and vigorously treat."

But while the problems for this patient may have been solved by the operation, the problem for another patient, who came to see one of the doctors two months later, was just beginning. This 24-year-old woman had no physical or emotional complaint, but simply wanted information about her risk of breast cancer and about health screening. The doctor examined her, and found nothing wrong except for a mid-systolic click—one of the signs of MVP—when he examined her heart.

The doctor ordered 24-hour electrocardiogram, echocardiography, and other tests. The echocardiogram showed an abnormality that was interpreted as MVP. A cardiologist recommended therapy with drugs to slow the heart rate, preventive antibiotics for dental and other procedures, semiannual monitoring for arrhythmias, and caution concerning overexertion. The patient was told that she suffered a disease of the mitral valve that could cause serious arrhythmias, other heart problems, fainting, or even sudden death.

Quite understandably, the patient and her husband became anxious. She worried about exercise, about being out of reach of emergency services, and whether it was safe for her to become pregnant and to raise a child. She started the drug to slow her heart, which made her feel emotionally flat and intellectually dull.

Distressed and uncertain, she was depressed for several months and worried about having a family. When she did become pregnant, she was considered at high risk, and was followed intensively through her anxiety-laden, but full-term normal pregnancy and delivery.

Meanwhile, her doctor was becoming skeptical about the so-called seriousness of MVP, and after her delivery he did not start her again on the heart medication. He later concluded that "the main risk of the many patients who have mild MVP is that of unnecessary medicalization."

PALPITATIONS AND ARRHYTHMIAS

Cardiology seems to be particularly full of terms that range from the trivial to the severe, leaving anguish and confusion in their wake. One of these terms is palpitations, which simply means that you can feel your heart beating; another is arrhythmias.

Arrhythmia means an abnormal heart rhythm and can range from manifestations of simple emotional disturbances to life-threatening disruptions of the heart's rhythm. The heart rhythm in fact is so susceptible to emotional factors that just taking the pulse of 225 patients in a coronary care unit significantly reduced their incidence of cardiac arrhythmias in the minute after the pulse was taken, showing how susceptible the heart is to human contact.

Arrhythmias, like murmurs and MVP, may be diagnosed simply because one is anxious about being in the doctor's office. But unlike the case of murmurs and MVP, the drug industry has played a role in promoting the dangers of arrhythmias, and there is no better example of interventions in which the risks of the disease were maximized and those of treatment minimized.

Here the tactic of choosing the wrong end point was used. As discussed in chapter 5, this consists of finding some marker or surrogate that seems to predict a bad outcome, treating the surrogate, and assuming that the outcome will be better. Researchers had found that when a certain type of arrhythmia, known as asymptomatic ventricular ectopic beats, was found in patients who had suffered a heart attack, these patients had an increased risk of sudden death. Doctors therefore reasoned that treating the arrhythmias would help prevent deaths, even though there was no evidence that this was so. Drug companies promoted the use of antiarrhythmic drugs, and from 1970 through 1986 the use of antiarrhythmic drugs by outpatients increased 200 percent. In the spring of 1989 I covered a symposium at Mt.

Sinai Hospital where the speaker, Mark E. Josephson, M.D., of the University of Pennsylvania, suggested that these drugs might be actually harming patients, and the reaction of the majority of the cardiologists present was shock: *not* to treat them would be malpractice, in the opinion of many of those present.

But the speaker turned out to be right. A few months later, the results of the Cardiac Arrhythmia Suppression Trial (CAST) study were published, showing that two of the drugs used to suppress the arrhythmias actually *increased* the death rate: patients treated with encainide and flecainide had nearly three times the death rate of those given a placebo! A third drug didn't increase the death rate, but it didn't decrease it, either. The arrhythmias in this case did predict a bad outcome, but treating them predicted an even worse one: many people who wouldn't have died otherwise were killed by their treatment.

But while some types of arrhythmia do predict a worse outcome, others seem to be totally benign, and sometimes even these are treated. In a recent survey, Dr. Joel Morganroth, of the Center of Excellence for Cardiovascular Studies at the University of Pennsylvania School of Medicine, found that 17 percent of cardiologists were treating arrhythmias that had absolutely no impact on health. This could be because the patients demanded it, but one wonders whether these patients had been adequately reassured that their arrhythmia was not dangerous and that the drugs they were taking to combat it possibly posed a greater risk. Dr. Josephson pointed out that if the goal of treating arrhythmias was to prevent symptoms, "First, I pat him [the patient] on the back and say not to worry and that works a fair amount of time. Then maybe I'll give him chewing gum, or whatever is the least expensive and least harmful [treatment] . . . just having the patient reassured and having them relax . . . is enough and the symptoms go away."

THE CASCADE EFFECT

The same type of arrhythmia treated in the CAST study has been found in 49 percent of normal, healthy elderly people, and James W. Mold, M.D., and Howard F. Stein, Ph.D., of the University of Oklahoma Health Sciences Center, cite the case of one lady in

whom it was discovered, terming her a victim of what they call
"the cascade effect—an initiating factor or factors, followed by a
series of events that seem to be direct results of previous events,
often catalyzed by some characteristic of the system—usually
anxiety."

This 81-year-old woman had been in excellent health and
completely independent and active when she was admitted to the
hospital with her arrhythmia, which was causing a mild degree
of congestive heart failure. She was started on four new drugs in
addition to the drug she was already taking for a hiatus hernia—
digoxin, quinidine, furosemide, and potassium, all for her heart.
She was discharged and readmitted two weeks later for digoxin
toxicity, which could have been predicted because digoxin reacts
with quinidine, and she was getting full doses of both drugs.

She was taken off the digoxin, but when this produced an
arrhythmia, she was started on an antiarrhythmic drug, tocainide,
and discharged from the hospital, still taking four different drugs.
Her symptoms of mental and physical deterioration—slowness,
difficulty thinking, and apathy—began shortly afterward. "One
can only speculate about the outcome had her original episode of
[arrhythmia] resolved before she was able to receive medical
care," the authors wrote. "We have been able to discontinue all
her medications except digoxin without any complications, and
her mental status seems to be improving gradually."

Obviously one solution here is for medical schools to give
future doctors better training in the art of reassuring well people
that indeed there is nothing wrong with them and in making the
treatment fit the illness in those who are slightly ill.

Dr. Stickler suggests that another very simple way to help
avoid labeling essentially healthy people with meaningless diagnoses is to change the forms on which diagnostic findings are
recorded. One of the problems, he says, is that when students are
forced to describe all the organ systems of patients they have
examined, they get bored writing things such as, "The abdomen
is soft, no masses can be palpated, and there is no enlargement of
the liver and spleen." According to Dr. Stickler, "Everyone knows
this dull litany and gets tired of writing or reading it. After the
tenth effort, the student is bound to find some enlargement

somewhere or hear some unusual noise over the heart or lung."

A form on which the physician need only circle or underline the various organ systems to signify that they had been examined and found normal would help, Dr. Stickler feels. "Perhaps most of us could teach brevity again and record only real abnormalities."

Chapter 12

The "Diseasing" of Risk Factors

High Cholesterol and High Blood Pressure

In an instant millions of Americans would acquire a dangerous condition that needed therapy under a doctor's supervision. . . . The world was learning how much money could be made scaring people about their cholesterol.
—Thomas Moore, *Heart Failure*, 1989.

If cholesterol had not existed, it would have had to be invented. Now some people are saying maybe it was.
—Russell Baker, *New York Times*, November 29, 1989.

Do all Americans brood about their cholesterol day and night?
All.
—Amanda Cross, *A Trap for Fools*.

Marianne Nestle, Ph.D., a nutritionist at New York University, collects horror stories about things that happen to people when they get their cholesterol measured.

One young woman she knows, for example, went to a clinic to obtain a prescription for the birth control pill. A few days later

171

she received a note in the mail that her cholesterol was 240 and the clinic could therefore not give her a prescription for the Pill. Nothing was said about what she might do about birth control, although a recommended diet was enclosed.

The young woman, understandably upset, phoned Dr. Nestle, who, familiar with the fallibility of tests for cholesterol or indeed most medical tests, suggested that the woman call the clinic and ask to be retested. The clinic claimed that its tests were accurate to 5 percent but nevertheless scheduled a retest. The young woman followed a low-fat, low-cholesterol diet prior to the test, but the second time around her cholesterol level measured 350.

Really upset now, she again telephoned Dr. Nestle, who made some inquiries as to the better testing labs in the city in which the young woman lived. The young woman took a third test, which came out 225, and was issued her prescription for the Pill. "What do you do?" she asked. "Keep getting it tested until you get one you like?"

When epidemiologists started studying the characteristics that make people more prone to heart attack and stroke, they started identifying "risk factors" such as high blood pressure, high cholesterol, smoking, and diabetes. Identifying such risk factors was useful, because it helped scientists understand something about how heart attacks and strokes developed and how they might be prevented.

RISK FACTOR MYTHS

But the two risk factors that were the most susceptible to being modified by drug therapy—high blood pressure and high cholesterol—soon came to be labeled "diseases" in themselves. From this labeling grew a whole infrastructure of national committees, specialists, and specialized centers—and the pharmaceutical companies that marketed drugs for high blood pressure and cholesterol—all having a stake in emphasizing their importance. There were several dramatic consequences to this:

- Risk factors have come to be seen as bad in themselves, even in situations where they are of very little risk to the people who have them.

- People assume that by treating the risk factors, they are preventing the disease for which the factors predict risk, which doesn't always prove to be the case.
- When there is no clear dividing line between who is normal and who is "high," the line is frequently drawn in such a way that the maximum number of people are labeled "at risk" and are therefore candidates for medical intervention.

As a consequence, many people are worrying about risk factors, spending money for testing for them, and even dying of the treatment for them, when these factors might better have been ignored, or at least kept in perspective.

- *Risk factors are promoted to diseases in themselves.* Consider the white woman who has high blood pressure (up to a diastolic pressure of 100) but doesn't smoke, has a normal cholesterol, and is not obese or diabetic. Her risk of having a heart attack or stroke is slightly higher than that of an otherwise comparable white woman without high blood pressure, but her absolute risk of having either a heart attack or a stroke is very low. While it probably wouldn't hurt for such a woman to adopt some kind of regular exercise plan, drug treatment is another matter; in fact, in the largest trial yet for the drug treatment of mild hypertension, women in this category who were treated with antihypertension drugs actually had a higher death rate than those treated with a placebo! There is little evidence that such women benefit from taking drugs for their high blood pressure, and since it usually produces no symptoms, drug treatment cannot be justified by the fact that it makes them feel better since it may actually make them feel worse.

Yet such women are usually treated with drugs in the United States, and in fact some hypertension specialists believe they are among the most treated, simply because they tend to be compliant patients. Because high blood pressure is more common in women (even though it is associated with such a low risk), some disease-mongers call high blood pressure a greater problem for women than for men, thereby totally dissociating the risk factor from the risk that originally defined it!

A similar situation pertains to white women with high cholesterol as their sole risk factor. "Women above the age of 50 have a higher mean cholesterol than men but a much lower risk of

CHD [coronary heart disease]," wrote S. G. Thompson and S. J. Pocock in the *Journal of Clinical Epidemiology.* "Other risk factors being equal, a woman with a high cholesterol level will have a substantially lower risk of CHD compared to a man with a much lower cholesterol level." While it might be better if these women's cholesterol were lower, their absolute risk of having a heart attack is still not very high. Like most labels, high cholesterol has vastly different meanings depending upon who has it. While a man who smokes heavily, is obese, doesn't exercise, and has high blood pressure and a cholesterol level of 300 and a slender, nonsmoking woman whose cholesterol is 220 may both speak about their "high cholesterol," this "disease" implies a vastly different risk for each. The man's risk of heart attack is high, and treatment may lower it significantly, resulting in a net benefit for him. The woman's risk is low, and there is a high probability that the treatment, and perhaps the label, will be worse than the "disease."

But disease-mongers tend to state that such complexities only confuse people, and "high cholesterol" became a disease based simply on the level of one's serum cholesterol, with the level at which it becomes a disease tending to get lower and lower. A release, for example, from the Vitamin Nutrition Information Service points out that high-risk serum cholesterol levels are most prevalent among women over 50 years of age, cleverly *not* pointing out that these women still have a lower risk of heart attack. A headline in the *New York Times* trumpets, "High Cholesterol Threatening Many: Study Says 80 percent of U.S. Males at Middle-Age Are Likely to Have Premature Death." Clearly it's an absurd oxymoron to say that 80 percent of men will have premature death, since a normal age of death is usually defined as the median age at which people die. Reading further in the story, we find that what it *really* says is that 80 percent of U.S. men were found to have cholesterol levels above 180 milligrams per deciliter (mg/dL) and that the risk of dying starts to go up above 180. According to the headline, this group is "likely" to have premature death—an enormous leap in logic.

- *Treating risk factors doesn't always reduce risk.* It was logical for the medical profession to assume that if high blood pressure and high cholesterol increased the risk of stroke and heart attacks, lowering both would reduce the risks. This worked for stroke, particularly for people with very high blood pressure: when people with high blood pressure were treated, their risk of stroke was lowered as much as their blood pressure.

But when the rate of heart attacks in the treated group was studied, observers were disappointed: bringing blood pressure down to normal didn't seem to cut the risk of heart attacks very much. In fact, the use of some types of blood pressure medications in some patients actually raised the death rate: a 1991 study performed at the Joslin Clinic in Boston showed that diabetics who also had high blood pressure had a higher death rate if given diuretic drugs for their high blood pressure than if their hypertension went untreated. Nobody knows quite how this happens, but diuretics tend to raise cholesterol, thus raising one risk factor in the process of lowering another. Another study published in 1991 showed that people taking any type of medication for hypertension increased their risk of becoming diabetic.

These findings caused some of the more thoughtful players in the hypertension field to rethink their assumptions, and they began to emphasize that the total risk should be evaluated, not the individual risk factors. If treating one risk factor had an adverse effect on the others, they concluded quite logically, they should then proceed with caution. "High blood pressure is not the problem," said Michael Alderman, M.D., of Albert Einstein College of Medicine in New York, in a debate held during the 1991 National Conference on Cholesterol and High Blood Pressure Control. "The problem is cardiovascular mortality. It's the absolute risk, not the level of blood pressure, that should be treated."

A similar dilemma haunted those looking carefully at the evidence that drug treatment of cholesterol was doing any good. High cholesterol, like high blood pressure, does increase the risk of having a heart attack. But when people whose cholesterol was very high were treated with cholesterol-lowering drugs and their survival was compared with people being given a placebo, two things became apparent. First, the drugs did seem to cut down on deaths from heart attack, although the magnitude of the reduction was quite mild. Second, in study after study there was no difference in the total mortality, because the deaths from heart disease in the group receiving placebo were always balanced by an increased death rate from something else—accidents, suicides, or cancer—in the groups receiving the cholesterol-lowering drugs.

As Tony Delamothe wrote in the British Medical Journal, "Most researchers agree that a raised blood cholesterol concentration is a risk factor for coronary heart disease, yet most agree that lowering people's blood cholesterol (either by diet or by drugs) does not affect their overall mortality."

Some studies, in fact, have shown more deaths in people treated for their cholesterol than in those not treated. At the end of a five-year trial in Finland, there was no significant difference in mortality between men who had been randomized to receive intensive risk-factor reduction including medication for both high blood pressure and high cholesterol or to a control group. But 10 years later, the group whose risks had supposedly been "reduced" had slightly more deaths than the controls—and significantly more deaths from cardiovascular disease, and from violence or accident.

Despite the fact that treating large numbers of people with expensive drugs and restrictive diets yielded such modest results, the NIH launched a National Cholesterol Education Program to get all Americans to know their cholesterol level and presumably to try to lower it—even though the NIH's own advisory council opposed such an emphasis in the face of such slight evidence. Eliot Corday, M.D., a clinical professor of medicine at the University of California at Los Angeles and a past president of the American College of Cardiology, was one of those advisers who in 1987 went on record in the New York Times as saying, "Why were they blowing this big program up that we could control cholesterol and reduce the mortality rate? We don't know what we're doing. It's absolutely ridiculous." In 1991 Dr. Corday confirmed that he had been accurately quoted and that he still stood behind his 1987 quote. "I feel the same, and so does a large segment of the medical profession," he told me.

Dr. Corday gave his own medical history as an example of why cholesterol manipulation doesn't help much. His own cholesterol had always been low, never going above 165, he explained. But his high-density lipoprotein (HDL) cholesterol ("good" cholesterol) was also low, and he eventually had a number of coronary complications requiring surgery. Dr. Corday agrees with many others that a low HDL cholesterol is a more important predictor of risk than total cholesterol. The problem, he says, is that it's difficult selectively to raise the HDL cholesterol: if you lower cholesterol, you lower HDL cholesterol, too.

Allan Brett, M.D., a general internist associated with Harvard Medical School, has analyzed the sometimes curious language used to explain the failure of anticholesterol drugs to bring down the death rate. The authors of one study, for example, "stated that 'the excess of deaths diverted attention from the principal study finding . . . [a lowered] incidence of coronary heart disease.' To consider an excess of deaths a diversion is to advance an odd point of view," Dr. Brett commented. He also pointed out that authors of another study dismissed the finding that people who took the cholesterol-lowering drug cholestyramine had a higher rate of violent and accidental deaths. "Since no plausible connection could be established between cholestyramine treatment and violent or accidental death, it is difficult to conclude that this could be anything but a chance occurrence." Dr. Brett notes that a similar trend occurred in another study, with the authors acknowledging that this trend "has also been observed in other studies" and then simply concluding that this outcome "has been interpreted to be a chance finding." Commented Dr. Brett: "The implication is that there are no precedents for the unintended behavioral effect of a medical intervention."

Social scientist Jonathan Cole has analyzed how scientists and the press distorted one of the major studies, the Lipid Research Clinics Coronary Primary Prevention Trial Results, to make the benefits of treating cholesterol seem much more important than the study actually showed.

In this trial, the study group of 1,906 subjects who received the drug cholestyramine for an average of 7.4 years was compared with the control group of 1,900 subjects who took a placebo for the same period, with both groups following a moderate cholesterol-lowering diet. Men in both groups had very high cholesterol levels. There were fewer deaths from coronary artery disease in the men receiving cholestyramine, and Cole points out that a typical headline for the study appeared in the *Los Angeles Times*, which said, "Cholesterol Decisively Linked to Heart Attacks."

The articles reported that the men had a 19-percent lower risk of having a heart attack and were 24 percent less apt to die of a heart attack than those who received only the placebo.

But, Cole points out, the stories failed to show that 38 of the control subjects died of heart attacks as compared with 30 of the subjects receiving cholestyramine, a difference of eight deaths from heart attack in 3,806 men over an average of seven years, which calculates to a death rate in the control group of 2 percent and a death rate in the study group of 1.6 percent. While, strictly speaking, the drop from 2 percent to 1.6 percent makes for a net reduction of 24-percent, it remains a drop of 0.4 of one percent, hardly an impressive difference. "Thus this major finding, hailed as definitive evidence of the harm of cholesterol, rests on this difference of 0.4 percent." The press rarely reported that (1) there was no difference in the death rates from all causes in the two groups and (2) that the men in the study all had very high cholesterol levels, so the results would not necessarily apply to people whose levels were lower.

Other studies have not shown much better results. Ralph Lach, M.D., director of the Adult Cardiovascular Training Program at Mount Carmel Medical Center in Columbus, Ohio, says, "If you take gemfibrozil [one of the cholesterol-lowering drugs] for a year, you have no greater chance of avoiding death and only a chance of one in 375 of avoiding any cardiovascular event. You do this at a cost of $700 to $1,000 a year. I don't think that if these figures were presented to the public anyone would take it."

As controversy continues about treating high cholesterol and high blood pressure, the disease-mongers have started looking at still another risk factor, high triglycerides. Stephen B. Hulley and Andrew L. Avins of the University of California, San Francisco, pointed out that the American Journal of Cardiology recently published a supplement about high triglycerides. The introduction had noted, correctly, that "the efficacy of reducing triglycerides to decrease coronary heart disease has not yet been conclusively established." However, Hulley and Avins pointed out, the concluding paragraph "ignores the controversy about whether drugs should be prescribed, instead advising physicians on which drug to use."

Dietary Therapy

Based upon the above information, some people might argue that, while perhaps the cholesterol-lowering drugs shouldn't be promoted, there's certainly no harm in trying to control cholesterol with diet. Most people agree that the American diet is high in fat, and we would probably be better off with less of it. Some people find that cutting down on fats has no negative effect on their quality of life.

But even here the health benefits are probably going to be very modest. W. C. Taylor and his associates from Boston, Massachusetts, developed a model that assumes cholesterol reduction is effective and safe in reducing the risk for death from CHD—in other words, giving the practice every benefit of the doubt because we don't really know what side effects may result after many years of cholesterol lowering. For persons aged 20 to 60 years at low risk, they calculated a gain in life expectancy of three days to three months from a lifelong program of cholesterol reduction. For persons at high risk, the calculated gain ranged from 18 days to 12 months. This was an average—some people's lives would be prolonged more, some not at all. Even in men who had already had a heart attack, where at least theoretically the benefit should be more than the risk, dietary advice saved one life a year—for every 9,000 heart attack patients given such advice. Another study found that if Americans could be persuaded to cut their fat intake from 37 percent of their total calories to 30 percent, the average life expectancy would increase three to four months, and most of the increased life would be for individuals over the age of 65. As Warren S. Browner wrote in the *Journal of the American Medical Association*, "If recent concerns about the possibly harmful effects of cholesterol lowering on mortality from noncardiovascular causes—which mainly affect younger persons—are valid, these relatively modest benefits would be overestimates of the actual effect."

For many people, cutting down on fats in their diet *does* affect the quality of life. "Many healthy, hungry men are worried, frustrated, and unhappy eating oat bran and rice bran, following diets without eggs, milk, butter, or red meats, and gorging on fish or the latest cholesterol-lowering fad food because they, their families, or even their physicians are convinced that immortality is ensured by unrealistically low serum cholesterol levels," wrote Dr. Hal B. Richerson, of the University of Iowa College of Medicine, in a letter to the *New England Journal of Medicine*. It's interesting that Sir Richard Doll, an English epidemiologist credited with first showing the relationship of smoking to lung cancer, of radiation to cancer, and many other correlations once said that he considered one of his greatest accomplishments was showing that people didn't have to go on bland diets for gastric ulcers. That finding, he said, "contributed to saving millions of people from having miserable diets imposed on them." Thomas N. James, M.D., a past president of the American Heart Association, was quoted in an article in the *New York Times* as saying, "One of the saddest things is to see patients who are in their 70s or 80s and who are terrified by what they are eating. One of the first things they want to know is what their cholesterol level is." Citing the fact that some elderly were even malnourished because they were afraid to eat their favorite foods, Dr. James said, "The obsession of the elderly with diet and cholesterol is a national tragedy."

Further Risks from Tests

With cholesterol testing, there may be a real negative side to the tests themselves, since not only are they inaccurate (which will be addressed in the next section), but they must be done with needles. Richard P. Kusserow, inspector general for the Department of Health and Human Services, told a congressional hearing in 1989 that some of the tests were conducted under unsanitary conditions by people who left bloody needles and specimens lying around, and some of the personnel gave tests and handled money without wearing rubber gloves or washing properly.

In addition, simply telling people their cholesterol or blood pressure is high can also have negative effects on their life. B. J. Milne and colleagues found that hypertensive subjects, both the newly labeled and the more established, scored significantly lower on many indices of psychosocial status—perception of health, total symptoms, worry, and the ability to participate in enjoyable activities—than did matched controls whose blood pressure was normal. R. Brian Haynes M.D. and his coworkers at McMaster University in Canada found that just telling people their blood pressure was high caused an 80 percent increase in absenteeism from work. Another study, which appeared in the *American Journal of Public Health*, found that people who had been told in the past that they had high blood pressure, but who had normal readings later, reported a worsening of their health over the past five years, even though by any objective measure their health had not worsened. Such findings should be a significant cause for concern in the light of the study reported in chapter 1 showing that people's own rating of their health predicted death better than most medical tests.

Dr. Brett, cites the case of a 61-year-old woman who went on a diet for her high cholesterol, lowering it to 251 mg/dL, but found that it went back up, despite continued dieting, to 281. This woman was already coping with a number of stressful events in her life, including the eviction of her elderly mother from an apartment, the divorce of her son, and the death of her daughter, in addition to the burden of worrying about her cholesterol levels. "She asked my permission to 'forget about her cholesterol,' because it had become the source of considerable anxiety in her daily life," wrote Dr. Brett. I once greeted a friend, asking him how he was. "Much better, thank you," he said, explaining that the improvement occurred after he had read my book *Medicine & Culture* and realized that his blood pressure wouldn't be considered serious enough to treat in Britain, even though his U.S. physician was treating it very aggressively. The book had given him reassurance that, at least by British standards, he was a well person.

In spite of such sobering evidence that the identification of risk factors is not always benign and ought to be kept in perspective, many doctors continue to believe that risk factors ought to be sought out and treated aggressively. One often-quoted advocate of treating hypertension at lower and lower levels, Ray Gifford, M.D., of the Cleveland Clinic, put it this way in a debate held during the 1991 National Conference on Cholesterol and High Blood Pressure Control: "How do you keep people in the system if you tell them they're O.K. and they don't need medication?"

- *The definition of who is sick is expanded.* If keeping people in the system and on medication is the goal, both hypertension and high cholesterol can be defined in ways that will include nearly everybody.

For example, if blood pressure is taken with the patient stressed, if the measurements aren't repeated, and if the cutoff of 140/90 is used as the level at which one should be treated, then a very large proportion of the population would be labeled as having high blood pressure. But if the blood pressure is taken as recommended after the patient has been sitting in a quiet room for five minutes, if it is taken at least twice on three different occasions, and if high blood pressure is defined as the level at which treatment has been clearly shown to be beneficial—a diastolic of 100 instead of 90—a dramatically lower number of people will be told they have high blood pressure and given drug therapy. Norman Kaplan, M.D., of the University of Texas Health Sciences Center at Dallas and author of *Clinical Hypertension,* estimates that the number of hypertensives cited in the population as 60 million would probably be lowered to about 40 million simply if the guidelines for taking blood pressure were followed, without even changing the level at which blood pressure was defined as high. Dr. Lach points out that one well-known study of hypertension therapy showed that drug treatment was clearly of benefit only in those people whose diastolic pressures were above 105. "But this would cut the number of people under treatment from 65 million to 2 million," which would bring a significant drop in profits for the relevant pharmaceutical companies. Those physicians who believe that risk factors should be treated in relation to the risk of disease would probably not accept a given number as the only criterion, but would treat according to the presence or absence of other risk factors. But with the growth of freestanding hypertension centers that exist only for the diagnosis and treatment of hypertension, there is a real incentive to diagnose low and to treat everybody.

A similar situation pertains to cholesterol. The National Cholesterol Education Program has defined the desirable cholesterol level as below 200, "borderline high" as 200–240, and "high" as over 240. Robert E. Olson, M.D., Ph.D., of the State University of New York at Stony Brook, points out that "borderline high" is already a contradiction in terms and that it's either borderline or high. And while doctors such as Dr. Olson believe it should be borderline, since a cholesterol up to 240 doesn't seem to pose much danger, there's a tendency to push it to high; indeed, a woman I know was given niacin for a cholesterol of 213, even though she had no other risk factors for heart attack. While the risk of cholesterol at this level is not great, niacin causes unpleasant flushing, and it has been linked to diabetes—a much more serious condition than a cholesterol level of 213.

In one recent report from Finland, for example, there was no increase in heart attack deaths among men who had serum cholesterol levels below 240 mg/dL and no evidence of heart disease. "Except to evangelists preaching that the lower the serum cholesterol level the better, the good news from the study is that levels below 240 mg/dL are all right for those without current manifestations of cardiovascular disease," wrote Dr. Richerson in his letter to the New England *Journal of Medicine*, "Yet, current recommendations for low-cholesterol diets to ensure longevity use 200 mg/dL as the desirable upper limit."

Furthermore, a single cholesterol reading is practically worthless. In 1985, the College of American Pathologists prepared a standardized blood sample with a cholesterol of 263 mg/dL and sent it to 5,000 laboratories. The reports came back with values ranging from 197 to 397, although the majority clustered in the range of 222 to 294. These widely varying readings were from laboratories; and cholesterol screening in malls is undoubtedly even less accurate. But besides the fact that different laboratories will measure exactly the same specimen differently, cholesterol will vary whether a person is standing up or lying down, according to season, whether a person has been exercising or losing weight, and whether or not the finger is squeezed during the procedure to help get the blood out, which 58 percent of technicians were found to be doing in public cholesterol screenings.

When people are advised to "know their cholesterol," the message is conveyed that the number is meaningful, leading to frustration when the cholesterol seems to rise from one reading to the next. Dr. Brett, for example, tells of a 33-year-old woman whose cholesterol was 205. Rather than tell her that this was a quite desirable cholesterol, as some doctors would have done, the doctor gave her dietary advice, and while her cholesterol was lower at the next reading, a few months later her cholesterol was 210, even though she was still following the same diet. "The patient was upset that 'my cholesterol is going up,' and she came to our office for a second opinion. Despite our efforts to assure her that her lipid profile was favorable and that it was common for cholesterol measurements to exhibit considerable variability, she remained obviously unsettled when she left the office."

In 1990, physicians reported treating serum cholesterol at considerably lower levels than in 1986 and 1983. The median range of serum cholesterol at which diet therapy was started was 200 to 219, down from 240 to 259 in 1986 and down from 260 to 279 in 1983. The median range for starting drug therapy was 240 to 259 in 1990, 300 to 319 in 1986, and 340 to 359 in 1983. Between 1983 and 1990, the number of adults reporting a physician diagnosis of high serum cholesterol increased from 7 percent to 16 percent, and the number reporting a prescribed cholesterol-lowering diet increased from 3 to 9 percent. Physicians around the country were invited to three-day sessions on the latest concepts about diagnosing and managing lipid disorders, with "lipid disorders" emerging as a clinical subspecialty.

The way in which disease-mongers continue to hype the risks of risk factors is especially evident in the way they evaluated one study designed to see if people could be screened for cholesterol and if they would see their doctor for follow-up if it was high. The study found that persons told their cholesterol was "high" were more likely to have seen their physicians three months later (50 percent) than those who were told their cholesterol was borderline (22 percent). Rather than simply accept this as rational behavior, as it would seem to most of us, the study's authors instead proposed hyping the risk even more: they suggested that the borderline category be eliminated in future screenings and that all participants who fell into the borderline category of 200 to 240 be told that their cholesterol was high!

Kiddie Cholesterol

It was probably only a matter of time until the cholesterol-mongers expanded to the only remaining segment of the population not already targeted: kids.

Kids don't have heart attacks (or if they do, they're very, very rarely due to occluded coronary arteries). But the disease-mongering theory says that the bad eating habits of children lead to high cholesterol in children, which leads to high cholesterol in adults, which leads to heart attacks. This view has been most strongly held by the American Health Foundation in New York, which has called for the screening of all children for high cholesterol. But three opponents of childhood screening ask readers to examine one paper making the case for such screening written by the foundation's director, E. L. Wynder, M.D.: "What they will find is a compilation of evidence suggesting that reducing children's cholesterol levels *might* [italics added] reduce their risk of future heart disease. What they will not find is any attempt to quantify how much the risk of heart disease might be decreased, how much it will cost to achieve that decrease, or how much the risk of other causes of death might be increased by cholesterol reduction," the three wrote. "It is dangerous to assume that the favorable effects of reducing cholesterol in middle-aged men can be generalized to children but that the unfavorable effects cannot."

Many thoughtful people believe that a lack of exercise and a junk food diet are probably not good for kids. But while exercise and a healthy diet should be encouraged (say, by getting McDonald's and other food providers to lower the fat content of their foods), it's another thing entirely to start measuring cholesterol levels in children and treating them with drugs. Not only would these children be "labeled" as having heart disease, but there's not even good evidence that children who have high cholesterol will have high cholesterol as adults. Ronald M. Lauer, M.D., and William B. Clarke, Ph.D., of the University of Iowa Hospitals and Clinics in Iowa City, determined that children with high cholesterol levels are very likely to become adults with desirable cholesterol levels without dietary or drug intervention.

But even if high cholesterol in childhood did predict high cholesterol in adulthood, it still wouldn't be a very good predictor of who will die from coronary heart disease. Assuming that those children who have high cholesterol in childhood will have it as adults, boys in the highest one-fifth of cholesterol levels have a 7.8 percent chance of dying of coronary artery disease before the age of 65, while boys with the lowest fifth have a 4.2 percent chance. In other words, the boys with the highest cholesterol levels are not even twice as likely to die of heart attacks before age 65 as those with the lowest levels.

Despite the uncertainty about the significance of cholesterol in childhood, the National Heart, Lung, and Blood Institute felt obliged to issue a statement on the issue. The statement itself was fairly reasonable (it gives the impression that people with widely divergent views on the matter had been locked up and forced to come to some kind of official consensus), with a call for healthier foods but also a statement that not all children need to be screened. The press conference held when the statement was issued was interesting since the various speakers of this so-called consensus were saying different things: officials from the institute said that high cholesterol in children predicted heart disease in adults, while Dr. Lauer, who also spoke, indicated that it didn't. More interesting, however, was the reaction of the press, or at least those attending the press conference. One man asked how many children were dying of heart attacks, which turned out to be an excellent question since the answers showed that high cholesterol in children was by no means an emergency. Others criticized the panel for not recommending national screening, seeming oblivious to the fact that our nation's children have many problems much more serious than cholesterol.

"Screening children, even the 25 percent with a family history of high blood cholesterol or early coronary artery disease, is a waste of money that is likely to do more harm than good," wrote Thomas B. Newman and his coworkers in the *Journal of the American Medical Association.*

But cholesterol is big business, both for the drug companies that sell cholesterol-lowering drugs like Mevacor and Zocor, which, combined, made $1 billion in 1990, and for the food companies that market foods low in cholesterol. "The cholesterol hysteria currently sweeping our country and its physicians is clearly the machination of the pharmaceutical industry," Dr. Ralph Lach wrote in *Ohio Medicine*. "It has funded a tremendous publicity frenzy that is not based in fact but which, unfortunately, takes advantage of a health-anxious public, well-intentioned but uninformed do-gooders and more-or-less willing physicians. The greatest gratification, however, is that of the drug industry which, according to some, stands to develop a 10–20 billion dollar-a-year business from its cholesterol scam."

Beyond measures like total abstinence from tobacco and maintenance of an ideal body weight through caloric restriction and dynamic exercise, "There is *no scientific evidence* that any further reduction of risk can be attained by any of the drugs, food products or 'low-cholesterol diets' being proposed so overwhelmingly," Dr. Lach continued. "The 'intertwining boards' have led to what amounts to a suppression of the negative view, even though the negative view is held by many authoritative figures."

Other physicians, such as Dr. Corday, twice president of the American College of Cardiology, have said that after they began to speak out against the National Cholesterol Education Program, they found their grant applications were being turned down.

What can be done? It's useful to look at what's happening in other countries. In Canada, for example, a working group strongly supported a general public health campaign to encourage community-wide changes in diet and life-style. It did not, however, recommend the universal screening of the adult population, and, as reported in the *New England Journal of Medicine*, cutoff points for intervention were set higher than those adopted in the United States on the grounds that "mass medicalization was not a sensible approach to a communitywide problem."

On a personal level, we can all start taking risk factors with a bit more skepticism. Avoiding mass screening programs is one way, since the results are likely to be inaccurate. Coupling risk factors to the diseases for which they predict risk is another: if your doctor says your blood pressure is high, try to pin him or her down on what your overall risk of heart attack or stroke is, and what the evidence is that by lowering your risk factors you'll decrease your risk. While the proverbial grain of salt may be bad for your blood pressure, it's definitely good seasoning to take with your medical information.

Chapter 13

The Medicalization of Menopause

Choose Your Disease

Every American woman should consider herself at risk [of breast cancer].
—Dr. Clark Heath, the American Cancer Society's vice president for epidemiology and statistics, *New York Times*, January 25, 1991.

Osteoporosis-related problems kill as many women each year as breast cancer.
—Press release, Wang Associates Health Communications. December 26, 1990.

Heart disease is the number-one killer of American women.
—Julia Kagan and Jo David, *McCalls*, June, 1991.

Because the disease-mongering machinery is fueled by as broad a target population as possible and driven by the apparent need for ongoing treatment, the ultimate disease-mongering scenario would be one in which the entire population would be convinced they need at least one pill a day for the rest of their life. Menopause may not be the ideal choice for this scenario, since it affects only women, but it comes close. In 1990, Premarin, a female hormone replacement therapy, was the fourth most prescribed medication in the United States, beaten only by an antibiotic, a heart medication, and an antiulcer drug.

How this natural life event, which affects every woman who lives long enough to reach it, has come to be seen as a disease to be treated won't be my main subject here, although it certainly fits into the category of medicalization. Through false analogy, this natural process is being treated as a hormone deficiency disease "like diabetes" or "like hypothyroidism." If women really benefited from medicalization of the menopause, I would be all for it. But rather than treat the more general issue of medicalization, I have chosen to deal with the issue pragmatically: Are women and their doctors getting the information they need to evaluate whether the benefits of taking hormone therapy are worth the risks?

The view being promulgated by many gynecologists, at meetings paid for by drug companies that manufacture estrogens, is that, indeed, the benefits are worth the risks, and all sorts of fantastic claims are being made for hormone replacement therapy (HRT), either estrogen alone or in combination with progestins. In a recent article in McCalls, for example, one researcher is quoted as saying that HRT adds four years to a woman's life and another, that the woman who has symptoms of the menopause is lucky because it gets her to the doctor's office, presumably for a diagnosis and prescription for hormone therapy.

But those promoting HRT are juggling several different effects of the hormones. On one hand, they relieve menopausal symptoms in some women, and they reduce the risk of osteoporosis. And some studies, none of them very good, indicate that HRT may reduce the risk of heart attacks. On the other hand, estrogens alone definitely increase the risk of cancer of the endometrium in women who have not had a hysterectomy, although the addition of progestins to the estrogens brings this risk down to normal. And a number of studies indicate that long-term use of HRT increases the risk of breast cancer; indeed, since many breast cancers grow under the influence of estrogen, it has long been suspected that they would.

Those promoting HRT for the "disease" of menopause follow a rather circuitous logic, saying that hormones don't cause breast cancer and that even if they do, these women are sent for mammography, and in any case breast cancer kills fewer people than heart disease, and HRT protects against heart disease. The New York Times coverage of the issue has been particularly pro-HRT, with the Times seeming to promote it even for women who've had breast cancer. In early 1992, for example, an analysis of a number of individual studies was published in the Lancet showing that several treatments for breast cancer, which had as a factor in common that they suppressed a woman's own hormones, all seemed to give women with breast cancer a better chance at survival. Yet Jane Brody (and in a similar article, Lawrence Altman) reported this story—which gives a strong indication that the particular hormones being currently used in HRT do promote the growth of breast cancer—with the curious statement that, after giving women treatments to suppress their natural hormones, "still unknown is whether it would be safe to give such women hormone replacements to relieve menopausal symptoms, reduce bone loss, and lower the risk of heart attack." It may be unknown in the sense that there have been no long-term trials where women who'd had their natural hormones removed in order to treat their breast cancer were given HRT, but the results certainly point to the fact that HRT would not be safe in these women.

But while the official viewpoint at meetings paid for by pharmaceutical firms manufacturing hormones is very pro-HRT, even at such meetings one finds dissenters who deserve to be taken seriously. At a cocktail party given at one recent international menopause meeting in Thailand, for example, I met a cancer expert from England who confided that he wouldn't let his wife take HRT because he wasn't certain that it didn't promote cancer. (His wife was one of those attractive older women whom ads promoting hormone therapy hint that you can be like only if you take HRT.)

Less anecdotally, there are some serious errors in the facts and reasoning of those who point out that HRT will be a boon to most women. The five most significant points, which I will explore in greater detail, are:

- The major trials of HRT to date have been nonrandomized and therefore subject to the serious bias that women who get hormones are generally more affluent and healthier than those who don't—and therefore would probably have a lower overall death rate in any case.

- The studies that show HRT may have a protective effect on the heart usually were made on women who were taking only estrogens. But most women are also prescribed progestins, which may negate the positive effects on the heart.
- Medical statistics do show that more women die of heart disease than breast cancer. But this is changing, with heart disease on the decline and breast cancer on the rise. And breast cancer kills at a younger age.
- The claim that women at high risk of breast cancer can be identified, and not given hormones, is highly suspect.
- While HRT helps prevent osteoporosis, other measures, such as calcium and exercise, can also be used against osteoporosis. Osteoporosis must to some extent be seen as a disease of medical progress, since it mostly affects people who have escaped early death from other causes, including breast cancer.

Let's look at these points in more detail.

- *Nearly all trials of HRT to date have been nonrandomized and therefore subject to serious bias.* The "gold standard" in clinical research is what is known as a randomized, controlled trial (RCT), in which people with the same degree of health or disease agree to be randomly allocated to receive one of two or more treatments, or sometimes a treatment or a placebo. The need for controlled trials was recognized at least as far back as the days of George Bernard Shaw, who wrote in the preface to The Doctor's Dilemma, "In Shakespear[e]'s time and for long after it, mummy was a favorite medicament. You took a pinch of the dust of a dead Egyptian in a pint of the hottest water you could bear to drink; and it did you a great deal of good. This, you thought, proved what a sovereign healer mummy was. But if you had tried the control experiment of taking the hot water without the mummy, you might have found the effect exactly the same, and that any hot drink would have done as well."

More recently, medical scientists tend to insist that to obtain sound answers to treatment questions, patients (or people) must be randomly allocated to (in other words, not allowed to choose) either the treatment or control group, to be sure that there are not subtle differences between the two groups that would influence the results of the trial. RCTs are not perfect: they tend to blur individualized responses, emphasizing populations instead. But they are the best standard to date of whether a given intervention is changing the natural course of the body in health or disease.

Researchers rely upon randomization because, if you compare people who chose one treatment with people who chose another treatment, you may encounter serious biases. For example, when breast-conserving operations for breast cancer were coming into vogue, scientists emphasized that you could not simply take women who chose to save their breasts and compare their survival with women who had mastectomies. Women who chose to save their breasts (or whose doctors decided were candidates for breast-conserving surgery) might differ in important ways from women who had mastectomies: their personalities might be different (one breast surgeon I interviewed suggested that they were crazy and therefore prone to live longer), or their breast lumps might be in some way less alarming. Breast surgeons in the United States were therefore categorically agreed that no lumpectomies could be done until the strictest standards of scientific proof were met. Similarly, the studies showing that low-dose aspirin can prevent heart attacks were randomized, with doctors randomized to take either aspirin or a placebo, and their rates of heart attack compared at a later date.

The importance placed on randomized, controlled trials in modern medical science makes it all the more shocking to realize that there has never been a long-term RCT comparing the outcome of women randomly allocated to take either HRT or a placebo, although one—widely expected to fail to produce a good answer because it is too complex—is planned by the National Institutes of Health. All the claims being made for HRT are being made on the basis of women who, with their doctor, decided for one reason or another to take, or not to take, HRT.

Let's consider what factors would make a woman and her doctor decide that she shouldn't take hormones. Since hormones are known to promote the growth of breast cancers, a woman with a history of breast cancer in her family would probably choose not to take hormones. It's therefore particularly alarming that a number of studies have shown an increased rate of breast cancer in women who take hormone therapy, since the women taking hormones are probably at a naturally lower risk for breast cancer than the general population.

Columnist Ellen Goodman, for example, gives an example of

how women and their doctors make such decisions. Two women, she says, saw their gynecologist for a mid-life checkup. Each woman shared her symptoms and her family history. Each received a thorough examination.

"One of this duo, however, left with a package of teeny-weeny hormone tablets, while the other did not. What made this surprising was that these women not only had the same complaints and the same doctor—they had the same family history. They were sisters."

The two later figured out that in fact they had given fairly different versions of their family medical history. "One emphasized cancer, the other did not."

Women with a family or personal history of heart disease probably also have, at least until recently, avoided taking hormones, since the similar hormones contained in the birth control pill have been associated with an increased rate of both stroke and heart attack. It's therefore not surprising that women taking HRT would have a lower rate of heart disease: they were probably at a lower risk to begin with.

Another factor indicating that women who choose to take hormones are healthier than other women is affluence. Wealthy women live longer than poor women, and this holds true regardless of whether rich women take HRT. Wealthy women are also more likely to take HRT because they can afford both the drugs and the visits to the doctor to monitor the effects of the drugs.

So women who have been taking HRT may well have been self-selected to have a lower rate of both breast cancer and heart disease and to be wealthier, and any claims made on the basis of current studies must take this into account. Only a randomized, controlled trial will resolve the question of whether HRT itself is influencing the rates of various diseases.

Epidemiologist Jan P. Vandenbroucke, M.D., of the University of Leiden in the Netherlands, pointed out, concerning one study widely cited as evidence that estrogen cut the death rate, that when women with preexisting disease were removed from the analysis, the mortality rates were similar in women taking, and those not taking, HRT. In all studies of estrogen substitution that are not randomized, he wrote in the Lancet, "it is still entirely possible that a woman who receives a prescription for hormone replacement is subtly healthier, or more determined to stay that way, than a woman who forgoes this therapy. Meta-analysis and cost-benefit analysis are unlikely to reveal the true benefits of oestrogen therapy if the increasing number of studies being pooled all have the same defect—ie., lack of comparability between users and nonusers. Perhaps we should demand some colossal well-controlled trials before we let the genie of universal preventive prescription escape from the bottle."

Another editorialist wrote in the Archives of Internal Medicine that the absence of reports from a randomized trial makes a recommendation to use estrogen in postmenopausal women "unjustified as a national public health policy." A study in the New England Journal of Medicine that was widely hailed as proof that women should take hormones was accompanied by an editorial that said, "There is always the lingering possibility that women who choose to take postmenopausal estrogens have other characteristics that explain their lower risk of ischemic heart disease. Only a randomized, controlled trial can effectively eliminate this potential bias. . . . The literature is replete with examples of randomized trials that failed to document the benefits suggested by less definitive study designs."

Despite this important caveat, Dr. Lee Goldman, who wrote the editorial, was quoted in the New York Times as saying, "The benefits of estrogen outweigh the risks, substantially." While the study fell just short of being "debate-ending," he expected that the results "will be a pendulum swinger,' leading many doctors and women who were undecided about whether to take estrogen after the menopause to take the hormone." These statements contrasted sharply with the more cautious—and scientific—tone of his editorial.

• *The studies that show HRT may have a protective effect on the heart looked only at estrogens.* In the summer of 1990, the FDA approved a label for estrogen therapy that claimed a protection for the heart in postmenopausal women without a uterus—an estimated 12 million U.S. women. As Fran Pollner wrote in Medical World News, this was based on a review of women who'd used estrogen replacement therapy. But none of the studies reviewed had also involved progestin, which is almost universally prescribed with estrogen for women who still have their uterus. Ezra Davidson, M.D., chairman of obstetrics and gynecology at the Charles R. Drew Postgraduate Medical School in Los Angeles, said that the drug's cardiovascular benefits were simply "presumed" and were not the "matter of science" that a committee vote implied.

This is a matter of some concern because progestins have an effect opposite to that of estrogen: chiefly that while estrogen can lower one's cholesterol level, progestins can raise it.

When a medical intervention causes a side effect, some doctors are always inclined to handle the side effect with yet another intervention, rather than using more caution in the first place. Some doctors, for example, now use the HRT argument to convince women to have hysterectomies, since a woman with no uterus can take estrogen without the added progestins.

• *Heart disease is on the decline, and breast cancer is on the rise.* It used to be that heart disease became the number one killer of women by about age 45, but the decline in heart disease—and the relative increase in deaths from cancer—has changed all this. A study reported by John Sutherland and his coworkers in the Journal of the American Medical Association showed that by about 1986, cancer had overtaken heart disease as the number one killer of both men and women under the age of 65. Not all the cancer in women is breast cancer; some of it's lung, colon, and other cancers. But in white women, breast cancer by itself is responsible for more years of potential life lost before age 65 than ischemic heart disease, the type of heart disease that might be favorably influenced by HRT.

Another factor that should be taken into consideration is that causes of death statistics are derived from death certificates, and studies that compared autopsy results with the cause of death given on death certificates have found wide discrepancies. Death certificates without autopsies are usually not all that accurate, and while death certificates are prepared for nearly everyone who dies, autopsies are performed only about 11 percent of the time. The inaccuracy isn't spread randomly but tends to affect some diseases more than others; several studies have shown that when people's death certificates say they died of a malignancy, they probably did. But a study by Constance Percy showed that when the person had a malignancy as well as some other condition, physicians in the United States were more likely than those in other countries to call the other condition the cause of death.

Ms. Percy wrote that a "problem arises when cancer is reported to be the cause of myocardial degeneration or coronary artery disease. U.S. coders assigned these deaths to the heart, whereas other countries tended to select cancer."

Deaths in the oldest age groups—where cardiovascular causes are cited by far the most frequently—are probably particularly suspect, since many people of this age have a variety of health problems and autopsies tend to be less frequent. Putting down "heart disease" on the death certificate may simply be a way to say that someone died of old age.

Some proponents of HRT claim that it hasn't yet been proven that HRT increases the risk of breast cancer. They say that the only study showing an increased risk of breast cancer was "the seriously flawed Swedish study"—always said with a high degree of xenophobia—failing to mention that while the study was carried out in Sweden, several of its investigators were from the U.S. National Cancer Institute. (One U.S. investigator wanted the "Swedish study" formally "denounced" at the 1989 North American Menopause Meeting, undoubtedly because it went against an earlier, much smaller study he had carried out.) In fact, an overall analysis of the studies on this issue indicates that long-term use (over 15 years) of HRT increases the incidence of breast cancer by about 30 percent—a sobering thought considering how common this cancer is to begin with. The Swedish study showed that adding progestins not only did not lessen the risk but might even add to it.

In addition, everything that we know about the biology of— and other risk factors for—breast cancer suggests that the more hormones (specifically estrogen and perhaps progesterone) that a woman produces naturally, the higher her risk of breast cancer. Early age of menstruation and late menopause, for example, increase the amount of hormones that a woman's breasts are exposed to naturally and have been found to increase the risk for breast cancer. Dietary effects on breast cancer risk might be mediated through hormones, since a high-fat diet produces higher levels of estrogen. Use of the birth control pill may increase the risk of breast cancer and may help explain why the incidence of breast cancer seems to be increasing. One of the first things a doctor does when a woman is diagnosed with breast cancer—at least if her cancer is hormone-receptive—is to try to shut off her natural hormones as much as possible. Some physicians, in fact, believe that the main effect of chemotherapy is to shut off hormone production, which is why it works better in premenopausal women than in women who have already passed menopause. All of this shows that there are both a theoretical reason hormones would increase the risk of breast cancer and some evidence that they are doing so.

Many women would probably choose, if they had to make a choice, to die of heart disease rather than of breast cancer, a death that often means pain and mutilation. Even if it is eventually proven that HRT prevents more deaths from heart disease than it causes from breast cancer, many women may still choose not to take HRT. Such women risk being labeled as "noncompliant" or irrational. One leading gynecologist, who admits that there is reason to believe that HRT will increase the risk of breast cancer, nevertheless sees the problem as one of compliance. "The issue is compliance, not cancer mortality. Protection against osteoporosis and cardiovascular disease requires long-term compliance, and fear of cancer is the problem, not cancer itself."

The risks of hormone therapy are dangerously underplayed in the way the message gets out to the general public as can be seen from the headline on a "Medical News Tips" press release from the Johns Hopkins Medical Institutions. The headline read: "Estrogen Replacement Therapy Safe," while the actual "tip" was more nuanced: "A clear-cut relationship between breast cancer and estrogen replacement therapy has not been documented," says Jean Anderson, M.D., assistant professor of gynecology and obstetrics at Johns Hopkins. "The evidence is still unclear." Now there's a significant difference between being innocent and being not proven guilty, and while human rights may say that people should be presumed innocent, there's no reason that drug therapies should, particularly considering past experiences that have shown that side effects don't emerge until years later. The blurb goes on to say that "estrogen replacement therapy is still the treatment of choice for most post-menopausal women," implying, of course, that menopause is a disease rather than a natural life event that the majority of women come through without major problems, living longer than men even without the benefits of drug treatment.

• *The claim that women at high risk of breast cancer can be identified and not given hormones is highly suspect.* Most women who get breast cancer do not have any risk factors for it. According to Susan Love, M.D., author of *Dr. Susan Love's Breast Book*, three-fourths of breast cancer patients don't. Ordering a mammogram before prescribing HRT may provide some legal protection for the doctor but little protection from breast cancer for the woman. Mammograms help only about one-third of women anyway, and they detect only cancers that have already been growing some six to eight years, a significant proportion of which will have already metastasized by the time they appear on the mammogram.

• *While HRT helps prevent osteoporosis, other measures, such as calcium and exercise, can also be used against osteoporosis.* More women are getting osteoporosis these days because they are living longer, and while it's certainly appropriate to try to improve their quality of life in old age, many women might prefer to try other means, such as calcium and exercise, until better data exist about the relationship between HRT and breast cancer. There may be better ways to prevent dying of osteoporosis-related causes at 80 than by dying of breast cancer at 60.

In addition, it bears reminding that the worst cases of osteoporosis tend to occur in women who have had their uterus and ovaries removed at a young age (and in people who take corticosteroid drugs), and this fact has been wielded by proponents of HRT to claim the protective effects of hormones. But there's another way of looking at this: it could be that nature provides the best protective system by giving women the benefits of hormones until about age 50 and then drastically reducing their amount. Medical scientists might assume, at least until the contrary is proven, that nature has its reasons. But in a society where a number of people stand to make more money by treating something than by not treating it, the side effects of an intervention are not taken as evidence that doctors should do less of the intervention; rather, they are taken as evidence that still another intervention is needed to combat the side effects of the first! The lesson disease-mongers drew from the past results of their interventions was not that they should intervene less but that "Estrogen is Good"!

DO WOMEN FEEL BETTER ON HRT?

When all else fails, proponents of HRT cite the fact that women feel better on HRT, so such treatment can be justified as a quality-of-life intervention. While it's true that many women do feel better, it's equally true that many women don't. If women always felt better, it would be hard to explain why doctors have so much trouble getting them to take hormones.

One doctor, for example, writing to the British Medical Journal about women who initially agreed to take hormones, found that a significant proportion of these women stopped taking them after one year primarily because of their side effects. By age, this group consisted of 6 of 16 women aged 40–49, 11 of 45 aged 50–59, 16 of 42 aged 60–69, and 3 of 6 aged 70 or over. In addition, 5 other women complained of symptoms that were not severe enough for them to cease treatment. Of the 19 women with an intact uterus, three complained about menstruation. Other common side effects in this age group included dizziness, headaches, cramps, and breast tenderness. Two of the women had phlebitis, and one had a deep venous thrombosis.

Proponents of HRT are confusing feeling good in the short term with preventing deterioration in the long run, and they are playing the two very different issues against women. When the inadequacies of the studies on long-term benefits are mentioned, HRT proponents counter that even if their long-term benefits haven't been proven, women feel better on hormones. When women complain about the side effects in the short term, they are told they should continue to take them anyway to prevent the long-term effects of their so-called hormone-deficiency disease.

Ann illustrates the difficult weighing of issues that women face when considering taking HRT. She stopped having her periods at age 45 but had no symptoms of the menopause. At age 46 she had an X ray for a knee problem and was told she had osteoporosis; she eventually saw an endocrinologist, who diagnosed a hyperactive parathyroid gland, a condition that leads to bone thinning, and she was told she had the bones of a 70-year-old woman. She had the parathyroid gland surgically removed and was advised to take HRT, at least for three years, to rebuild her bones. She had heard good things about HRT: that it would keep her vagina and eyes lubricated and that it might prevent heart attacks. There had been no breast cancer in her family, and her father had had a number of heart attacks, so she looked like the ideal candidate for hormone therapy, even to physicians fairly conservative about prescribing it.

But while she was taking HRT, she gained weight, and her breasts began to grow, from a C cup bra to a DD cup. While she thought these changes were simply due to the aging process, she also developed lumps under her arms and eventually saw a breast surgeon, who said that the lumps were not cancerous but probably due to the stimulation of the breast tissue there by the HRT, probably the progestins. Ann asked if she could take estrogen without progestin, and the breast surgeon responded in the negative. She also asked if she could take a lower dose of HRT and was told there was no evidence that a lower dose would help her osteoporosis.

Not wanting to be crippled by osteoporosis, but not wanting to be crippled by constantly enlarging breasts, either, and wondering what effect such stimulation would have on her risk of breast cancer, she told the endocrinologist that she wanted to discontinue the hormones. Her endocrinologist did not oppose this decision, noting that "most people would rather die of heart attacks than of cancer." The endocrinologist prescribed another treatment for osteoporosis, but was somewhat abashed a few months later when studies showed that this drug actually increased the severity of osteoporosis rather than decreasing it. Ann discontinued the hormones and found that the weight she had gained on HRT miraculously came off, and her breasts became softer, with the lumps under her arms disappearing. A few months later her younger sister, 46 and premenopausal, was diagnosed with breast cancer, thus increasing Ann's perceived risk of getting breast cancer herself.

Women taking HRT today are participating in a vast experiment, and the risks and benefits of treatment remain to be known. As participants in this experiment, they deserve better information about the uncertainties involved than they are getting.

Chapter 14

"Precancerous" Breasts and the Overselling of Mammography

'Cancer will never be cured unless the medical profession starts a *cancer panic*,' Dr. James Coupal, President Coolidge's personal physician, said here. Dr. Coupal deplored the tendency of physicians today to hush up both the rates of incidence and the effects of the disease in an effort to minimize its horrors in the eyes of the public. '*Cancerphobia* must be inculcated into everyone over 31,' the doctor said.
—*International Herald Tribune*, August 22, 1928.

FIBROCYSTIC BREAST DISEASE

In 1986 the College of American Pathologists held a press conference on so-called fibrocystic disease, a term used to describe many different, benign conditions of the breast. There was no free lunch to attract reporters, as is usually the custom for such events (not even coffee that I recall), and the conference was not well attended.

The poor attendance and the consequent scarce publicity were unfortunate, because the pathologists had called their conference for the purpose of de-mongering a disease. Fibrocystic breast disease, they declared, is not in fact a disease at all and usually is not even a risk factor for breast cancer.

This doesn't mean that women who have fibrocystic disease don't sometimes get breast cancer; it just means that they seem no more likely to get it than anybody else. Susan Love, M.D., a breast surgeon from Boston, has most consistently let the way in pointing out that fibrocystic disease is a meaningless label, and that it harms women.

A few years before the 1986 press conference, Dr. Love had written an article for the *New England Journal of Medicine* titled "Fibrocystic 'Disease' of the Breast—a Nondisease?" As Dr. Love pointed out in her article, one doctor doesn't know what another doctor is talking about when they talk about fibrocystic disease, and most women with fibrocystic disease—some 90 percent of women—have no higher risk of breast cancer than do the other 10 percent who have no fibrocystic disease. Fibrocystic disease simply means lumpy breasts, and lumpy breasts, while harder to examine than nonlumpy ones, are normal. Dr. Love, speaking to a Women and Cancer Conference in New York in 1985, said, "What you consider a disease as opposed to normal is very subjective, and has no hard-core basis in medical practice. Some breasts feel like a cobblestone road: some feel like gravel."

As Dr. Love sees it, surgeons (with the cooperation of pathologists) use the term as a convenient catchall when they've done a biopsy and don't want to tell their patients they haven't found anything. When radiologists use the term, it usually just means that the woman is young and has the normally dense breasts of a younger woman. "Dense breast tissue is in fact very normal, especially in young women. There's nothing diseased about it, except in the imaginations of some doctors."

Of course, for women whose breasts are painful, treatment to relieve their pain might be justified, although Dr. Love points out that a lot of the pain is related to the fear that they have cancer or at least are at a higher risk for it, and simple reassurance is probably the best treatment. Some women find that limiting coffee, tea, and other foods such as chocolate that contain the substance xanthine seems to help. But controlled trials, in which the examiners didn't know which women had been on the special diets, found no difference in the actual texture of the breasts of women who had followed the special diets and those who hadn't.

It would thus appear that the diets work mostly by the placebo effect, perhaps by relieving women's fear that they are at special risk of cancer. Dr. Love calls a caffeine-free diet one of the bigger hoaxes put over on women—although if it makes you feel better, then you should by all means try it.

But heavier and more invasive treatments are also frequently advised. Some doctors prescribe danazol, a drug that causes acne, weight gain, and generally a severe masculinization; some even advise bilateral mastectomy, or removal of both breasts, which they justify to other doctors as being recommended because the woman seemed pathologically afraid of cancer, although these doctors rarely look at where—or from whom—their patients may have gotten that fear. Sometimes the bilateral mastectomy is performed as a subcutaneous mastectomy, whereby most of the breast tissue is removed and replaced with an implant under the skin. Such an operation, while possibly good from a cosmetic standpoint, doesn't eliminate the risk of breast cancer, since there is still some breast tissue left. It makes the breasts almost impossible to examine mammographically, and it adds all the hazards of breast implants.

While the condition it seeks to describe may be harmless, and the term itself is meaningless, fibrocystic disease is dangerous. As Dr. Love wrote in her recently published *Dr. Susan Love's Breast Book*:

> Many insurance companies won't insure a woman who's been diagnosed as having fibrocystic disease—as they won't insure people diagnosed as having any chronic disease. If they'll insure you at all, they may exclude breast problems— with the result that you won't have insurance coverage should you ever get a real breast disease.
>
> At the same time, if you're already insured when you're diagnosed as having fibrocystic disease, your company may pay for your mammograms. Because of this, a well-meaning doctor is often tempted to diagnose fibrocystic disease so your mammogram will be paid for. But your advantage then lasts only as long as you remain with the same insurance company: should you ever want to sign up with another company, your "disease" will work against you, and you'll be stuck with the label for the rest of your life.

So this is definitely a diagnosis you should try to keep off your medical records, since it doesn't mean anything, yet can work against you. As we saw in chapter 1, there's no rhyme or reason as to what insurance companies will and will not insure, and the myth of fibrocystic disease gets them off the hook. Since all women are at a reasonably high risk of breast cancer, and breast cancer costs insurance companies more than any other disease, the meaningless diagnosis of fibrocystic disease is just an excuse for them to exclude women or to exclude coverage for their breasts. If a doctor tells you that you have fibrocystic disease, try to tell him or her that you do not want this on your record and explain why. (You might try showing the doctor Dr. Love's article, which appeared in the *New England Journal of Medicine*, vol. 307, no. 16, October 14, 1982, pp. 1010–1014.) Many states now make it mandatory that companies pay for screening mammograms, and you don't need a diagnosis for a screening mammogram. If you don't live in one of these states, and your doctor tries to use the diagnosis of fibrocystic disease to get insurance coverage for your mammogram, think twice about submitting that insurance form. One hopes that in a few years this diagnosis will be recognized as the nonsense that it is.

THE OVERSELLING OF MAMMOGRAPHY

"THIS WOMAN JUST MISSED THE CANCER THAT WILL KILL HER," trumpets the ad for the Mammography Center in Ontario Community Hospital, Ontario, California, showing the picture of a seemingly young woman examining her breasts. The text says that while the woman cannot detect Stage 0 breast cancer, mammography can.

Advertisements like this create the impression that no woman need ever die of breast cancer if she simply has mammograms often enough. As an article in the *Journal of the National Cancer Institute* points out, "Campaigns for early detection implicitly promise that regular mammograms and physical (including self-) examinations can avert serious illness and death from breast cancer." The reality is somewhat different. Early detection can cut deaths from breast cancer by about one-third in women over age 50, but won't affect the other two-thirds. In younger women the benefits are even less—if they exist at all.

In fact, ads like the one above have less to do with public health than with the fact that hospitals have so overbought mammography equipment that even if every woman for whom mammography was recommended had the examination at the recommended interval, there would still be "excess capacity." U.S. hospitals, doctors' offices, and diagnostic centers have two to four times as many mammography X-ray machines as are needed for screening and diagnosis, creating a scramble for potential patients; what's more, only one-fifth of the machines are accredited by the American College of Radiology! According to Robert McLelland, M.D., of the University of North Carolina School of Medicine, even "some primary care physicians have been doing the procedure in their practices. Stated reasons include convenience, increased patient compliance, and lower costs, but there are probably profit motives as well. This is incredible in view of the complexities and difficulties in doing high-quality mammography even by well-trained and experienced personnel."

Mammography machines are expensive, and in order to recoup the investment and make them pay, doctors must either charge more money per mammogram or perform more mammograms. One way to perform more mammograms is to try to get more women over the age of 50 in whom mammograms have actually been shown to cut the death rate from breast cancer, to get the recommended number of mammograms, since there are still a sizable number of women who do not. But another way is to cater to the health conscious younger woman, for whom no responsible group is recommending screening mammograms because they are useless and potentially dangerous. As an article in the journal *Cancer* put it:

> The evidence for the usefulness of mammography in screening women for breast cancer varies with age. For women aged 50 to 74 years, the evidence is strong, and there is universal agreement among expert groups that these women should receive regular mammography. For women in their 40s, the evidence is less clear, and expert groups disagree in their screening recommendations. For women younger than 40 years of age, the low incidence of breast cancer and the low sensitivity of mammography have led to a consensus that routine screening with mammography is not indicated. Few groups now recommend even a "baseline" mammogram for women younger than 40 years of age.

But while screening mammography is useless in young women, many of the advertisements do not acknowledge this and seem, in fact, to be catering to the younger audience. One recent ad widely broadcast on television, for example, says that the sponsoring company has developed a technique that makes mammography safer for young women, failing to acknowledge that the problem in young women is not simply safety but the fact that mammograms are unlikely to show cancers—or, indeed, any tumors at all—in their dense breasts. The cynicism underlying the ads, in fact, is witnessed by the fact that at the same time General Electric was aggressively advertising mammography on TV, it was not paying for screening mammograms among its own employees, even though it was in a state (Connecticut) that made such payments for screening mandatory. After *Connecticut* magazine pointed this out, GE changed its policy.

But the ads seem to be working. As the article in *Cancer* noted, a substantial percentage (19 percent) of physicians said that they ordered "regular screening mammograms" on 81 to 100 percent of their 30- to 39-year-old women patients, and 15 percent of women in the same age group had had a mammogram within the previous year.

OVERESTIMATING THE RISK

While the lifetime risk of breast cancer is fairly high, with a woman's having a 1-in-9 risk of developing it if she lives to the age of 110, some surveys have shown that women vastly overestimate their risk of being diagnosed in any given year or on any mammogram. One survey of New England women, for example, found that 16 percent thought there was a 1-in-10 chance of having a breast cancer found on the mammogram, and 26 percent thought there was a 1-in-100 chance, a risk from 4 to 600 times the actual age-specific incidence of breast cancer at ages 30–60. In actual fact, at age 40, the chance of having breast cancer diagnosed in a given year is 1 in 1,200, and at age 50, 1 in 590; even at the highest risk, age 80, the estimated incidence is 1 in 290.

This fear has been fueled by pronouncements of the American Cancer Society, which promulgates the lifetime risk of 1-in-

9 without clarifying that the risk in a given year is much less. Sandra Blakeslee, writing in the *New York Times*, quoted an American Cancer Society spokeswoman as saying "The 1-in-9 is meant to be a jolt. . . . It's meant to be more of a metaphor than a hard figure." According to I. Craig Henderson, M.D., director of clinical cancer programs at the University of California at San Francisco, quoted in the same article, "They may have botched it. In their enthusiasm to help women, they created an epidemic of fear."

Physicians, he said, are adding to the problem because they are not trained in statistics and sometimes add up the "risks" in preposterous ways, telling women that their risks are not 1-in-9, but 1-in-2.

As a consequence, some women become so fearful of breast cancer that they have their healthy breasts removed to avoid getting cancer, often in the operation known as subcutaneous mastectomy in which an implant is inserted under the skin after most of the breast tissue has been removed. As John E. Woods, M.D., and Phillip G. Arnold, M.D., of the Mayo Clinic, wrote in response to a recent article in the *Wall Street Journal*, "It is from women who literally live in terror of breast cancer because of high risk that the impetus for the procedure comes." Another correspondent, Vincent R. Pennisi, M.D., of St. Francis Memorial Hospital in San Francisco, citing the fact that the death rate from breast cancer was going up, wrote that "every surgeon should offer a woman who is at high risk the option of prophylactic mastectomy."

Breast cancer rates are indeed going up, but at least some of this increase is due to what scientists refer to as artifacts. One such artifact is that with techniques such as mammography, some of the cancers found are really precancers that would, in the absence of mammography, have stayed in some women's breasts all their lives until they died of something else. With widespread screening, doctors are picking up those tumors that in former years would have eventually surfaced, but they're also picking up a large number of precancers, making the number of people diagnosed with cancer seem larger without there necessarily being more cancer. (Besides making it appear that cancer is increasing, this phenomenon also makes it appear that cure rates are going up, since precancers are easily "cured.") Another is that more women are living longer, and since the risk of getting breast cancer increases with age, more women are getting cancer. This phenomenon accounts not only for some of the increase in the number of people diagnosed with cancer, but also for some of the increase in people dying of cancer. Breast cancer rates probably really are increasing, and certainly it's becoming a more important cause of death as deaths from heart disease are decreasing, but the numbers cited often make the increase appear greater than it really is.

Many people would say, "Why shouldn't young women have mammograms if there is any chance at all they would detect breast cancer? After all, young women occasionally do get breast cancer, and these cases are particularly tragic." The answer is that there are significant downsides to mammography:

- Mammograms often don't find cancers in the dense breasts of young women. Even if they do, the evidence is not strong that such women will live longer than they would have if they'd waited for the cancer to surface before going for treatment, although they might have a better chance of breast-conserving surgery.
- Mammograms detect other, ultimately benign abnormalities that doctors feel they must check out, resulting in anguish and unnecessary surgery and expense.
- Some women find mammograms painful.
- While the risk of radiation-induced cancer in a woman who starts getting mammograms at age 40 or 50 is not felt to be high, the risk of a woman who starts in her twenties will be much higher.

Let's look at these points one by one.

- *Mammograms often don't find cancers in the dense breasts of young women.* During a recent call-in show addressing the issue of breast cancer on National Public Radio, a woman who had a strong family history of breast cancer said that she'd had her first mammogram at the age of 21, at which time "hyperplasia" (cellular proliferation) was diagnosed. Her sister hadn't had a mammogram and had died of breast cancer at age 27. She'd often wondered what would have happened if her sister had had a mammogram in her twenties, as she had.

Dr. Love, one of the panelists on the show, was blunt: "It

wouldn't have found the cancer, that's what would have happened." Dr. Love further explained that the woman's diagnosis of hyperplasia was simply a result of having a mammogram at age 21, with the dense breasts that young women normally have being interpreted as disease.

Dr. Susan M. Williams, a radiologist at the University of Nebraska Medical Center, writing in the journal *Radiology*, reviewed the mammograms of 76 women aged 18 to 29 who were referred to her because they had lumps in their breast. In 74 percent the mammogram did not even show the lump, and in the other cases the X-ray examination did not in any way change the patient's treatment.

While the lumps in these very young women were not cancerous, mammography will often fail to show even breast cancers that are large enough to be felt. Stanley Edeiken, M.D., of the Jersey Shore Medical Center in Neptune, New Jersey, sent all his female patients with suspicious lumps for mammograms and later for biopsy. Overall, one-fifth of the women who were found on biopsy to have cancer had had negative mammograms, and in the 50-and-under age group, 44 percent of the cancers did not show on the mammogram. "These studies demonstrate that the false-negative rate is much higher than usually reported in the literature and that mammography is far less sensitive than reported to the public," he wrote in the journal *Cancer*.

Ferris M. Hall, M.D., of the department of radiology at Beth Israel Hospital and Harvard Medical School, wrote in a letter to the journal *Radiology* that when a woman schedules a mammography examination, his department asks her age, and if she is under 30, the physician who requested the mammogram is asked to talk with the radiologist. The radiologist tells the woman's doctor that (1) breast cancer in this age group is uncommon, (2) the mammogram is likely to convey less information and to require more radiation for penetration because of the normally greater density of breasts in women in this age group, and (3) radiation in younger women is proportionally more carcinogenic. This advice is obviously in the woman's interest, but it's not likely to happen when people are trying to capitalize on their mammography equipment.

Mammograms are based on the fact that cancerous tissue has a density different from that of the normal breast, which tends to be true when you're over age 50, but less so when you're age 25. "A mammogram in a woman in her twenties will show absolutely nothing, because women that age have dense breast tissue," said Dr. Kathleen Mayzel, associate director of Boston's Faulkner Breast Centre. "At around age 35 we start getting fatty replacement in our breasts," so that mammograms may begin to detect cancers.

Between the ages of 35 and 50 there seems to be a mixed situation, as some women still have dense breasts, and others have less dense ones. So a woman in this age group has a better chance of getting a mammogram that actually tells something. It's also true that about one-third of breast cancers are diagnosed between the ages of 39 and 49 and that breast cancer is the number one cause of death in women this age.

But even with a better chance that mammography will be helpful in women age 40 to 50, trials comparing the death rate from breast cancer in women who had regular mammograms compared with women who didn't haven't shown much difference. The same four randomized, controlled trials that showed that women over age 50 benefited from mammograms, with a death rate about one-third lower than the rate for those who didn't have mammograms, showed no immediate difference in the death rate in women age 40 to 50. One study, done by New York's Health Insurance Plan (HIP), did tend to show that about seven years after the screening started, women who had been screened by both mammography and physical examination started to have a lower death rate from breast cancer than women who didn't get either. On the basis of this one study some groups in the United States now recommend that women age 40 to 50 get mammograms every year or two.

But the evidence that mammograms help in this age group is still very weak. None of the other three studies has shown any benefit of screening by mammography in women under age 50, and the New York study was a study not just of mammography, but also of physical examination, and it could be the physical examination that is making the difference. One ongoing study in Canada, in fact, where women who receive physical examination and mammography are being compared with those who receive physical examination alone is showing that women who get the additional mammography have a *higher* death rate from breast cancer than those getting just physical examination. Many people cannot explain why the women getting mammograms would have a higher death rate from breast cancer. But the evidence that it helps is so poor that most other developed countries—and some groups in the United States—recommend that screening start at age 50.

Many people I talk to simply cannot understand how it could be possible that mammography would detect some cancers, yet not change the death rate from breast cancer, given the barrage of propaganda about early detection that we have been given. It's true that mammography tends to detect small cancers, and it's true that women found to have small cancers usually have a better outcome than those with large cancers. But a cancer can be small for one of two reasons: either it's been found early, or it's a very slow-growing, not very aggressive tumor. Screening usually detects a large proportion of the latter, and some of these would probably not ever have killed the woman anyway.

A particular case in point is those cancers called *in situ* cancers, meaning that they have not yet started to invade the surrounding tissue. Mammograms are particularly good at picking up *in situ* ductal cancers, and so the incidence of cancer is rising partly because these "precancers" are being detected and called cancer. In the past, in situ cancers made up about 5–10 percent of all breast cancers, but with increased use of mammography many more of these "early" breast cancers are being found, and now about 20 percent of detected breast cancers are "ductal carcinoma in situ" (DCIS). As Dr. Love wrote in the *Harvard Medical School Health Letter,* "Before mammography came into wide use, we thought DCIS was very rare. It didn't form lumps, and at that time we were operating only on lumps. So we missed it—or if we found it, we removed the breast. But now that so much screening mammography is being done, we're finding DCIS all the time."

If these precancers are detected and called cancer and the woman treated as if she had cancer, the outcome is likely to be favorable. But even if they hadn't been detected and treated, only about one-third of these would ever have become invasive cancers. One study of consecutive autopsies done in Denmark found that of 77 women who'd died of other causes without ever knowing they had breast cancer, one had invasive cancer, and 14, or 18 percent, had in situ cancers. A woman may very well want to have such a cancer detected, particularly if it can be removed with minimal disfigurement. But detection of in situ cancers may not have much impact on the death rate as a whole, since the majority of these women wouldn't have died of their cancer even if it hadn't been detected.

The other reason mammography doesn't have much impact on survival figures in the under-50 age group is that mammography is not really early detection: it detects cancers that have been growing for about six years. Many of the invasive cancers detected will already have spread by the time they are detected by mammography, and since it is the metastases that ultimately kill, treatment will already be too late.

One recent book on breast cancer, for example, included a chapter on how doctors can defend themselves in court if sued for not finding a breast cancer. Two of the defenses mentioned were the "doubling time" defense and the "so-what" defense. In the discussion of the "doubling time" defense, the writers go over the math necessary to convince a jury that a cancer big enough to be found by physical examination has had to be growing in the patient's breast for nearly 8 years. "Based on these scientific facts, the argument can be advanced that the tumor is more likely to have metastasized before the alleged negligent act than during the alleged delay between the defendant's first opportunity to diagnose and the time that the tumor was finally diagnosed." The "so-what" defense is similar, showing that by the time a lump is palpable, there's also a significant possibility that the cancer has metastasized.

While mammography *may* (but certainly doesn't always) find a cancer one to two years before it would be palpated, the cancer has still been there a long time, and the same defenses would apply.

The overselling of mammography is extremely prejudicial to women for two reasons: since everyone assumes that breast cancer can be prevented, any woman who gets it anyway is considered negligent, though even in the age groups where mammography works best, it cuts the death rate only by about one-third. A negative mammogram gives doctors a false sense of security. As Caroline A. Jones wrote in a letter to the *New York Times*: "Among the 14 or so young women in my breast cancer support group, only one had her lump identified by a mammogram. The rest of us, having identified our tumors ourselves, were sent away by surgeons waving 'clear' mammograms." One series of 52 cancers in patients under age 45 showed that the mammograms were initially reported as negative in 33, or nearly two-thirds of the patients. In 15 of the patients, this resulted in a delay of biopsy. Even more shocking is the fact that mammography is often used to justify practices that might, in fact, increase a woman's chances of getting breast cancer, such as hormone replacement therapy. Since mammograms are not early detection, using them to say it's all right to give women drugs that may increase their risk of breast cancer is frightening.

• *Mammograms detect noncancerous abnormalities that must be checked out, resulting in anguish and unnecessary surgery and expense.* In any large-scale screening program, the proportion of mammograms interpreted as abnormal is as high as 15–20 percent. Most of these women do not have breast cancer; they just have abnormal mammograms.

This percentage translates into an enormous number of women: if 45 percent of the 48 million American women 40 years of age or older had yearly mammograms, the estimated number of abnormal mammograms would be more than four million per year, and the proportion is even higher in younger age groups. The mental anguish that an abnormal mammogram can cause is considerable: 17 percent of women with highly suspicious findings indicated that their ability to engage in their daily activities was compromised, and 26 percent indicated that their moods were affected even after breast cancer was subsequently ruled out. The people who performed the study were not worried about the functioning of these women, however, only about whether they would continue to get mammograms.

Women with abnormal mammograms are usually sent for biopsies, a minor surgical procedure, but nonetheless costly and carrying a slight risk. Because radiologists are afraid of being sued for not recommending a biopsy, they will tend to recommend one on the slightest suspicion of abnormality. As an article in the *Journal of the National Cancer Institute* noted, "Observers have questioned to what degree biopsy recommendations may be motivated by physicians' fear of malpractice suits rather than by their wish to offer patients optimal care." According to Martin A. Thomas, M.D., a veteran mammographer who practices in Washington, D.C.: "When I started performing mammography, we felt that a diagnostic radiologist should recover a cancer in about 1 of 3 biopsies that he recommended." Now many radiologists recommend biopsy when there is even the slightest possibility of cancer, meaning that only one in 20 biopsies show cancer. "My own diagnostic criteria for recommending biopsy have changed dramatically in the last 2 or 3 years, and a lot of that has to do with not wanting to get sued." In some cases, U.S. doctors may recommend biopsies for a level of suspicion that is even lower. As a Lansing, Michigan, doctor wrote in the October 17, 1990, *Journal of the American Medical Association*, "Unfortunately, a 1 to 100 chance of cancer must be an indication for biopsy [considering] that . . . deciding not to obtain a biopsy specimen could easily result in a million-dollar judgment against the physician who made that call."

American women undergoing screening for breast cancer are more likely to be referred for surgical biopsy than their counterparts in several other countries. Figures from one center in England, for example, showed that rather than recommending 20 biopsies for every one cancer, which is the American average, the British radiologists in 1991 recommended a total of 23 biopsies, of which 21 turned out to be cancers.

Maureen, an editor in her early fifties living in a southern city, was referred to a surgeon when a screening mammogram showed a small lump just under her breast. The surgeon wanted to hospitalize her immediately for a biopsy under general anesthesia. But Maureen recalled that about seven years ago, in another city, someone had found a lump in the same place on her mammogram and told her it was probably scar tissue from an earlier breast reduction operation.

Maureen suggested to the surgeon that she call for the earlier mammogram, which could then be compared with the current one; if the lump was the same size, in the same place, then no biopsy should be necessary. The surgeon's response was strange: he advised her not to bother "because it would only cause us not to operate." Maureen obtained the earlier mammogram anyway and consulted a radiologist specializing in cancer, who found that the current lump was exactly the same size and in the same place as shown on the mammogram taken years earlier, and therefore it was extremely unlikely to be a cancer. She *didn't* have the biopsy.

Such a low threshold for recommending biopsy can result in a large number of women having a breast biopsy at some point in their life. Margaret found that having had two previous breast biopsies worked against her getting insurance. When her Blue Cross payments became too much for her budget, a little investigation showed she could get a better rate with Mutual of Omaha. Because she had had two previous biopsies, however, her contract specifically stated that the insurance would not cover anything concerning her breasts for several years.

• *Some women find mammograms painful.* This issue has probably been most thoroughly dealt with in the "Letters to Ann Landers" newspaper column. In order to perform a mammogram, the breast is squashed between two plates, and depending on the skill of the technician and the pain sensitivity of the woman, it may be simply uncomfortable or so painful that the woman faints. Ann's answer is that it's always worth it to prevent breast cancer, but, as we have seen, only in the women over age 50 is there clear-cut evidence of any drop in the death rate from breast cancer attributable to screening mammograms.

• *While the risk of radiation-induced cancer in a woman who starts getting mammograms at age 40 or 50 is not felt to be high, the risk of a woman who starts in her twenties will be much higher.* The larger and denser a woman's breasts are, the higher the dose of radiation necessary to get a good mammogram. Since young women have dense breasts, they'll be given a higher dose. Not only will the dose be higher, but a woman who starts getting mammograms at age 20 will be getting many more of them over her lifetime, and the risks of radiation accumulate with every dose.

In addition, because the growth of the mammography industry has been so rapid, the regulators are not able to ensure that all equipment is of the highest quality. Dr. McLelland, chairman of the American College of Radiology's Committee on Breast Imaging, was quoted as saying in the *Journal of the National Cancer Institute*, the oversupply of mammography equipment "is further aggravated by an aggressive industry willing to promote and sell the equipment to anyone regardless of qualifications, resulting in the use of machines that are not accredited or regulated in any way." While more than 30 states have laws requiring insurance reimbursement for mammograms, only two include comprehensive standards for quality assurance.

Dr. Coupal's aim of starting a cancer panic, noted at the beginning of this chapter, has clearly succeeded, with women now greatly overestimating their chances of getting breast cancer in any given year. Yet in spite of the fact that more women are examining their breasts, going to their doctors, and getting mammograms than ever before, the death rate from breast cancer has actually increased in the United States over the past 40 years. Many people are still trying to blame women for the increase: women may have been examining their breasts in record numbers, but they do it wrong; they may have been going for mammography, but not often enough. They are told that they are getting more breast cancer because they are having their children later, for while teenage pregnancy is a social problem, it does help prevent breast cancer; or they are told that they get breast cancer because they eat too much fat, even though Dr. Love points out that women are now eating less fat (and getting more breast cancer) than they did a century ago. Public pronouncements often leave the impression that breast cancer could be wiped out if only women could be panicked enough into cooperating.

But the evidence says otherwise. Use of high-quality mammograms in women over the age of 50 could, in fact, cut the death rate from breast cancer, but only modestly, and even women who do everything right still have a significant risk of dying of breast cancer. It's time to shift our focus away from blaming the victims to looking at where the money's going in the fight against breast cancer and who's profiting: it's *not* all those young women getting mammograms.

Chapter 15

Cosmetic Considerations

I believe that we are in the midst of an alarming rise of hucksterism, a fearful professional pestilence. Subtly or blatantly, many plastic surgeons and many who are nonplastic surgeons but who do our work are not offering their skills, but are peddling a product—and not primarily to aid the patient as much as to help themselves.

> —Robert M. Goldwyn, M.D., *Plastic and Reconstructive Surgery*, February 1989.

There is a substantial and enlarging body of medical information and opinion . . . to the effect that [the female breast that does not achieve normal or adequate development is] really a disease which in most patients result in feelings of inadequacy, lack of self-confidence, distortion of body image and a total lack of well being due to a lack of self-perceived femininity.

> —H. William Potterfield, past president of the American Society of Plastic and Reconstructive Surgeons. Quoted in the *Wall Street Journal*, March 12, 1992.

When Brenda took her eight-year-old son to the dentist, the dentist told her that the boy should see an orthodontist for braces because he was "tongue thrusting"—pushing his tongue against his teeth, causing the teeth to move slowly outward. The dentist told Brenda that her son's tongue thrusting was causing his teeth to become maloccluded, or misaligned. In addition to getting braces, the dentist recommended that the tongue thrusting itself be treated, since the teeth would otherwise become maloccluded again after the braces were removed.

Brenda couldn't see anything particularly wrong with her son's teeth, and she found the term "tongue thrusting" both comic and slightly salacious, but she dutifully took her son to an orthodontist. When she asked what her son risked if he didn't get braces, she was told in a vague way that it might be important later on. While not really satisfied with the answer, she nevertheless decided that her son should have the braces. "You're more vulnerable when your children are involved," she explained later. "You might accept something less than perfect for yourself, but you think, 'This child has the potential to grow up perfect. He'll probably get the Nobel Prize, and when he goes up on stage . . .'"

But the orthodontist caused her son considerable pain when he first put the braces on, something she had not expected and which she resented since, after all, she was doing this for her son's sake. The orthodontist then told her the braces would have to be tightened every two to three weeks, causing days of chronic pain each time, and handed her a warning sheet about how important it was for someone with braces to brush correctly, causing her to worry when her son had gone to bed and she wasn't certain he'd remembered to brush his teeth. "I was not told these things before the braces were put on his teeth," Brenda recalled. The original dentist wanted the braces removed at the twice-yearly dental examination. This meant that every six months Brenda had to take her son to the orthodontist to remove the braces, to the dentist for the checkup, and back to the orthodontist to put the braces back on.

"It was a hideous, hideous inconvenience," said Brenda, who was working full-time and had a younger son at home. "In the final analysis, they scare you—that's why you do it." Since her son didn't wear a retainer because he kept losing it, after the braces were removed for good, his teeth seemed to move slowly back to their original position.

Brenda tried to find someone to correct the tongue thrusting, but was told by a speech therapist that he would work only with someone whose speech was affected, and her son's speech was not. Her dentist didn't persist in his original advice, however, and soon seemed to forget about the tongue thrusting , which was by that time falling out of fashion as a diagnosis.

Dr. Peter S. Vig, a professor of orthodontics at the University of Pittsburgh, chuckled when I asked him about the diagnosis of tongue thrusting. Tongue thrusting, he explained, is a normal developmental phase that most children grow out of. "It was big as a diagnosis in the 1950s and again in the 1970s, and now it's big in Switzerland because the dentist promoting it moved there," he said.

There's nothing wrong with doctors' and dentists' performing procedures to improve someone's appearance, and indeed many medical interventions are purely cosmetic. Minimizing the scarring of someone who's been in an accident, reconstructing a breast following mastectomy, and correcting serious cosmetic birth defects probably do a lot more to help people than many other medical interventions that are performed purportedly to lengthen life or to improve function. But the number of cosmetic surgeons has increased even faster than the number of other physicians, quadrupling in the past quarter century. As Boyd R. Burkhardt, a Tucson-based plastic surgeon, was quoted in the *New York Times* as saying, "There are only so many head injuries, so many cleft lips and palates. The one expandable part of the territory is cosmetic surgery." Many procedures done by dentists, orthodontists, dental surgeons, dermatologists, ear, nose, and throat surgeons, and even gynecologists must ultimately be justified on cosmetic grounds. If you cannot convince people they are sick, you can convince them that they are ugly—and perhaps that their ugliness qualifies as "disease."

Mongering procedures for purely cosmetic considerations can be insidious in at least three ways. The first is when a condition is most often purely cosmetic but can occasionally be associated with other problems and the doctor—sometimes in collusion with the patient, who is trying to get insurance coverage—exaggerates the other problems. The second is when the cosmetic defect is so subtle that the patient hasn't been bothered by it until told by the doctor that he or she has "a disease," usually with an impressive Latin or Greek name. The third is when both patient and doctor know that the procedure is being done for purely cosmetic reasons, but the doctor minimizes the risks of the procedure, thereby distorting the information that the patient needs in order to make an informed choice.

EXAGGERATING PROBLEMS

As an example of the first mongering procedure, take malocclusions, which orthodontists frequently correct. Eighty-five percent of malocclusions are purely a question of esthetics, and should be seen as such. As Dr. Vig wrote in a recent book titled *Current Controversies in Orthodontics*, "A number of studies in facial attractiveness are claimed to have validated the hypotheses of 'Anatomy is destiny' and 'Beauty is good.' Social adaptation and chances for success are apparently improved by facial attractiveness. In contrast, the evidence for any causal relationship between malocclusion and poor oral health is weak." Occasionally, says Dr. Kitty Tulloch, an orthodontist at the University of North Carolina at Chapel Hill, teeth that stick out too much can break more readily.

But dentists and orthodontists don't always explain to the patient that malocclusion in the vast majority of cases is just a question of looks. When I first started seeing New York dentists, for example, they didn't seem to notice anything abnormal about me until I opened my mouth. But they would check my "bite," which one dentist diagnosed as "terrible," and he told me I had "severe malocclusion." "Do you have trouble eating?" he asked, a question that is quite amusing to anyone who knows me well, since I am one of those people who live to eat. Since the dentist had no way of knowing this, I asked him if I looked malnourished. While he agreed I didn't, he was still ready to refer me to an orthodontist. When I persisted in asking about the disadvantage of my "severe malocclusion," the dentist suggested that perhaps I would have more difficulty eating a steak than he would, admitting that perhaps in a world where steaks are considered bad for you this might actually be an *advantage*.

While it's easy to accuse orthodontists of wanting to make money, the puzzle here is that in both Brenda's case and mine it was the referring dentist who suggested orthodontia, and unless they were receiving illegal kickbacks, there was no direct benefit for them.

"I think it's the way dentists are trained," said Dr. Ronald Strauss, of the Department of Dental Ecology at the University of North Carolina at Chapel Hill. "In dental school you're taught how to recognize the four stages of malocclusion," and just assume they all need to be corrected. "Historically," wrote Dr. Vig, "orthodontists have laid greater emphasis on mastering their art than their science. Educational establishments have stressed the how rather than the why, where, or when."

"Unlike other health-care specialties," he went on, "no aspect of orthodontics has yet been evaluated to yield any data on efficacy." In other words, no one knows whether orthodontia actually works, even when "working" means only improved appearance. "Orthodontists rarely see their patients several years after completion of treatment to be able to assess the long-term success of their particular orthodontic intervention."

Orthodontics is only one of many specialties that claim to be treating "disease" but that must ultimately justify many of their interventions strictly on the basis of improving appearance. Dermatologists refer to acne as "a disease," but it's only of cosmetic importance and often goes away on its own; in addition, dermatologists remove various lumps and bumps because they could be "precancerous," without clarifying how likely this is or whether there's any risk waiting until it does. Ear, nose, and throat surgeons frequently "fix" deviated septa of the nose, which are mainly cosmetic problems, and probably not even that unless you often have people in a position to be looking up your nostrils. Ophthalmologists may not level with patients that while their drooping eyelids *may* impair vision, they don't always do so, and fixing them if they don't is purely a cosmetic operation. Cosmetic surgeons often justify breast reduction operations on the grounds that the breasts may be so heavy they strain the back or that the woman is psychologically distressed about having large breasts, which may or may not be true.

While gynecologists often tell women that large fibroid tumors of the uterus may be cancerous or may damage the kidneys, if you point out that both these conditions are relatively rare, they'll often fall back on the argument that large fibroids can cause the abdomen to bulge. The practice of describing the size of a uterus with fibroid tumors in terms of months of pregnancy—"Your uterus is the size of a six-month pregnancy"—is one way of making the cosmetic defect sound worse than it really is. Such a uterus may extend *up* to the belly button, just as does the uterus of a woman who is six months' pregnant. But it usually doesn't extend *out* nearly as much, and the woman will probably not look as if she is six months' pregnant. While gyne-cologists in this country almost uniformly recommend hysterec-tomy for a fibroid uterus greater than the size of a three-month pregnancy, a Swedish gynecologist I spoke to said he would not perform a hysterectomy on a woman whose uterus was the size of a six-month pregnancy unless she was complaining of symp-toms and wanted the operation for that reason.

Another reason gynecologists use to justify hysterectomy is that women with heavy periods may stain their clothes, and one southern gynecologist told me, "Since I live in the South, I have girls who tell me in the summer they're afraid of wearing white dresses because they bleed through them and that's socially handicapping. And if that's a real bother to them, then I think doctors need to be concerned in trying to fix it whatever way they can." If both doctor and patient understand that being able to wear white clothes is the only issue, this is perhaps acceptable. But one woman I know was told *after* her hysterectomy by her gynecologist, "Aren't you happy to be able to wear anything you want now?" The woman was shocked that her doctor could even consider this important enough to *talk* about.

CONVINCING PEOPLE THEY ARE UGLY

The second way that doctors can monger their procedures is by admitting that certain procedures are done for purely cosmetic reasons, but by making patients feel that they have a greater cosmetic defect than they did before they entered the doctor's office. Before a dermatologist told me that I had "acne rosacea"—a condition that means basically that I flush easily—it didn't bother me at all, and, in fact, my friends complimented me on my good color, telling me that I didn't really need to wear makeup. After the diagnosis, I began to feel self-conscious and was less likely to go out without makeup. (I rejected the cortisone cream that the dermatologist prescribed, however, since it was purely symptomatic and might have made my face worse if I'd used it very often.) A study in Holland compared patients' perceptions of whether they needed cosmetic dentistry with dentists' perceptions, and while up to 40 percent of patients thought they needed interventions, the dentists judged that up to 63 percent did. Dr.

Robert Goldwyn, editor of the *Journal of Plastic and Reconstructive Surgery*, knows of cosmetic surgeons who, when patients come to see them for a procedure such as scar removal, will tell them, "I think you would look better with a nose job," thereby subtly—or not so subtly—eroding their self-image. Indeed, the offices of many plastic surgeons seem calculated to make the normal person feel inadequate. When Jane Berentson, pursuing a story for the *Wall Street Journal*, presented herself as a candidate for implant surgery, she found that "the ambiance is more beauty parlor than doctor's office, with mirrors everywhere and plenty of good-looking assistants, one of whom helpfully opened her blouse, unhooked her bra, and pointed out the barely visible scar from her own saline-implant surgery."

Playing into this is the notion, promoted by cosmetic surgeons, that there is some absolute, unvarying standard of beauty against which they can judge all women (and, increasingly, men), while in fact standards of beauty have varied over time and across cultures. The ideal female body used to be short and positively dumpy as judged by today's standards, and the ideal breast size in France and most of Europe is much smaller than that in the United States: while most cosmetic breast operations performed in the United States are augmentations (130,000 each year), in Europe the majority of cosmetic operations on the breast are *reductions*. As Dr. Vladimir Mitz, a Parisian plastic surgeon who has worked in the United States, said, "Many breasts reduced in France would be considered very beautiful in America before they were reduced." Dr. Vig recalls picking up an issue of *Vogue* and realizing that many of the models could be considered to have "long-face syndrome" and/or "skin grin" (excessive gingival display), conditions that he and his colleagues were correcting—on the basis that they were cosmetic defects—in the late 1970s and early 1980s.

As the level of medicalization in a country increases—usually due to an increase in the number of doctors—lesser and lesser "defects" are treated with more and more aggressive procedures. According to Dr. Strauss, "A child who may have been acceptably 'bucktoothed' in the 1940s and who may have been a candidate for orthodontic braces in the 1950s and 1960s now often has a 'dentofacial deformity,' the treatment for which is maxillofacial surgery. The expansion of medical attention toward this nonlife-threatening condition serves to increase its unacceptability as normal. As a result, a minor variant of normal becomes a deformity." Dr. Strauss points out that, just as a surgeon can make people think they are more deformed, "a statement from a surgeon that a condition is not serious enough to operate on may be interpreted as a certification of physical acceptability and normality." But the number of oral-maxillofacial surgeons increased from around 1,500 in 1965 to nearly 4,000 in 1980, a trend that mitigates against such statements.

MINIMIZING THE RISKS

The third mongering procedure is minimizing the risks. Doctors who treat conditions other than purely cosmetic ones may sometimes confuse the issue of whether proposed treatment is based on cosmetic considerations or "disease"; but most people who go to cosmetic surgeons know that they are there to try to look better, not to live longer. And to make an informed choice about whether they want to undergo surgery to try to look better, they need particularly clear information about the risks of treatment. But if the case of silicone implants is any indication, many are not getting the full story.

At this writing, nobody knows how dangerous silicone implants are or were, but that is just the point: for 30 years women were told that they were safe in spite of the fact that nobody had any information on their safety and there were reports of problems. As a result of this apparent campaign of misinformation, well over a million American women underwent breast implant surgery, 80 percent of them for purely cosmetic reasons. Marsha Chambers, for example, a 44-year-old Tustin, California, woman, was quoted in the *New York Times* as saying, "My doctor told me that even though it was dangerous to inject silicone, these were in bags, so there was no risk. He said the silicone couldn't come out unless my chest got crushed in a car accident, and ha, ha, ha, how often does that happen?" The FDA didn't require any data until very recently, and the manufacturers put off collecting them. As Sidney M. Wolfe, M.D., director of the Public Citizen Health Research Group, wrote in a letter to the *Wall Street Journal*, "One of the most well-documented problems caused by silicone-gel breast implants is interference with mammography," which, at least in women over age 50, could delay the diagnosis of breast cancer, leading in turn to a lower chance for a cure. "Interestingly, human studies with alternative implants, filled with absorbable, metabolizable vegetable oil that does not interfere with mammography, have been delayed because companies such as Dow (the chief manufacturer of silicone-gel implants) would not support such research, so long as they can keep selling silicone-gel implants," Dr. Wolfe wrote. Plastic surgeons claimed that they didn't see problems in women getting the implants, but they seem to have forgotten that a patient who develops rheumatism several years after her implant would see a rheumatologist rather than a plastic surgeon, so that in fact they had no way to follow up their patients.

According to Joan E. Rigdon, writing in the *Wall Street Journal*, when reports started surfacing that the implants might be dangerous, the people who made the reports were vilified. When Dr. Frank Vasey, a Florida rheumatologist, published a paper that implants might trigger autoimmune disorders, some local plastic surgeons held a press conference in Tampa and blasted him for "filling up [medical] journals with garbage." Many plastic surgeons, according to the *Journal*, failed to alert women to possible health risks reported by several sources, including professional journals, manufacturers, and some of their own patients. The American Society for Plastic and Reconstructive Surgery—considered one of the more responsible of the associations of plastic surgeons—collected millions of dollars from its members to lobby to keep the devices on the market and, even when the controversy was at its hottest, maintained a hotline giving patients statements about implants that, according to the FDA, "overstate the safety of breast implants and minimize known or suspected side effects." When Jane Berentson presented herself as a patient to four New York cosmetic surgeons during the time the silicone implants were banned, none of them mentioned that the saline-filled implants they were recommending might also interfere with mammography and might possibly cause autoimmune diseases or cancer.

Unlike breasts that are "too small" or "too large," some cosmetic "problems" will go away on their own and may be made worse if you try to treat them. Strawberry birthmarks, often found on children, may sometimes be troubling from a cosmetic standpoint, but are usually better left alone, says Gunnar B. Stickler, M.D., former chairman of the department of pediatrics at the Mayo Clinic, since in most cases they will eventually disappear by school age, and attempts to remove them will often leave permanent scars. A woman I know who was given several drugs for her diagnosis of acne rosacea, one of which was supposed to be used only for life-threatening conditions, decided instead to throw away the drugs and cured her condition—later diagnosed as "cortisone burn" by another dermatologist—by switching to a mild soap and hypoallergenic cosmetics.

IS SHORTNESS A DISEASE?

While I had never been troubled by malocclusion or acne rosacea and indeed didn't know I had either condition until doctors told me so when I was consulting them for something else, I have always been short and acutely aware of all the disadvantages of it: being treated as if I were a child, getting stepped on because people don't see me, having trouble finding clothes to fit, not being able to reach things on the shelves, and, perhaps the worst, not being able to eat as much without getting fat. If there were exercises to grow taller, I would probably do them, and when I contemplated having a child I seriously considered how to go about finding a tall father. Most of my short friends—I'm talking about women around five feet tall—feel the same way, and a lot of us cringed when the film director Roman Polanski was overlooked by the emcee at a recent awards ceremony at the Cannes film festival and referred to by a disgruntled director as "the midget."

But none of us believes that the answer lies in treating normally short children with shots of human growth hormone, a treatment that gives uncertain results and costs $15,000 a year. We ourselves would not take it if that were still a possibility, nor would those of us who have children want our children to take it.

For one thing, there is no evidence that it works in the normally short, other than producing a transient growth spurt that may not lead to an adult height any greater than the person would have reached without it. And the treatment brings potentially serious side effects. The first people so treated were given growth hormone extracted from the brains of corpses. Initially, it was thought that the only adverse effect of this treatment was the formation of antibodies to growth hormone, which rarely inhibited the response. But as in so many other medical interventions, people simply hadn't waited long enough for the side effects to appear. In 1985 it was discovered that some of these people had acquired a slow virus disease known as Creutzfeldt-Jakob disease, which leads to dementia and death. Doctors have subsequently stopped using the natural human growth hormone and now use one that is synthetically made, and it should be safer.

But nobody knows enough about how the normal body works to know what the long-term side effects will be. One study in England found that children given growth hormone became skinny, "with obvious loss of adipose tissue from all areas of the body but especially from the limbs and face. The girls in particular looked inappropriately muscular." These researchers found that the initial growth spurt seemed to be fueled by stored body fat and suggested that the growth spurt may stop because the stored fat is used up. It's probably much safer and certainly cheaper for those of us who are normally short to get into some kind of therapy, posture training, or instruction in high-authority dressing, if necessary. Perhaps we could carry boa constrictors to make people notice us, as does La Toya Jackson, although I'm not certain the long-term side effects of this are well known!

What's most insidious about the promotion of human growth hormone treatment, to those of us who are short, is that to sell the treatment, the company marketing the hormone has to sell normal shortness as "a disease" rather than simply an inconvenience—a "postural deficit," as one official of the company that makes the synthetic growth hormone described in a letter to the editor of the *New York Times Magazine*. That makes us feel worse than we did before.

"Until growth hormone came along, no one called normal shortness a disease," Dr. John D. Lantos, of the Center for Clinical Medical Ethics at the University of Chicago Pritzker School of Medicine, was quoted as saying in the *New York Times Magazine*. "It's become a disease only because a manipulation has become available, and because doctors and insurance companies, in order to rationalize their actions, have had to perceive it as one. What we're seeing is two things—the commodotization of drugs that are well-being enhancers and the creeping redefinition of what it means to be healthy."

But I would argue, as one of the normally short, that to refer to such drugs as "well-being enhancers" is premature and too kind. Until there are much more data about both the efficacy and the side effects of this treatment of the normally short, the promotion of shortness as a disease is more serious than simply a creeping medicalization; rather, it's another blatant instance in which a "disease" is sold to the American public based on an underestimation of the risks of treatment and the overselling of its benefits. Even if it were safe and worked, treating the shortest people would simply raise the average height level of the population, creating a whole new class of "short" individuals who would now be 5'2" instead of 4'11"!

The medicalization of "shortness" takes a particularly insidious turn when normally short infants are diagnosed as having the condition "failure to thrive" simply because they are smaller than other infants of the same age. Dr. Stickler says that this term is used for a variety of conditions, including some that may be serious, such as dwarfism, or failure to gain and to grow. "In our practice," wrote Dr. Stickler, "we see with increasing frequency short infants considered to have failure to thrive. There seems to be a pattern: they undergo a multitude of diagnostic tests. Suspicions are even raised that the parents are child abusers who are not providing enough food or love or both. In the absence of specific findings, these children are put through various feeding schemes. The mother may have been breast-feeding, and she is the first to be blamed for not having enough milk. The infant is given a prepared cow's milk formula, and when this does not work, milk allergy is suspected and the child is given a soy-based formula." Commonly, says Dr. Stickler, parents and doctors will try to force more calories into the child by inserting a feeding tube into its stomach, which may make the child start vomiting. The vomiting is then "fixed" by an operation that tightens the connection between the esophagus and the stomach.

Dr. Stickler cited the case of a boy he first saw at age 19 months who had such a feeding tube in his stomach, which caused the child to vomit occasionally. The child looked well, however, and Dr. Stickler learned that one of his maternal aunts was only 4'9" tall and that his two grandmothers were 4'10" and 5'1" tall. Although the parents were reluctant to have the feeding tube removed, they allowed it to be clamped and eventually removed. The boy continued to grow and had no further vomiting or feeding difficulties.

But as the long-term side effects of various procedures done primarily for cosmetic purposes become manifest, resulting in curbs on their use, new "cures" for new "diseases" take their places. At the same time that some doctors question whether normally short children should be treated with shots of human growth hormone, others have begun to advocate shots of the same hormone to build muscle mass in older people. Enthusiasm about the treatment was sparked by a study in the *New England Journal of Medicine,* and newsletters devoted to the hormone started up, as did referrals to Swiss clinics where the hormone is prescribed for about $23,000 a year. Follow-up studies that indicated treatment benefits were temporary and side effects, including water-weight gain, carpal-tunnel syndrome, and enlargement of male breasts, failed to generate headlines, according to Marilyn Chase writing in the *Wall Street Journal.*

And just as the possible risks of some 30 years of breast augmentation were being publicized, at least one cosmetic surgeon was promoting penile augmentation, known more "scientifically" as circumferential autologous penile engorgement. "Who am I to decide if a patient's penis is large enough?" the surgeon performing the operations was quoted as saying in *Omni* magazine. "This procedure dramatically improves self-esteem."

The same benefit was, of course, the reason so many women underwent breast implant surgery: the risks of such surgical solutions to self-esteem remain unknown.

Chapter 16

Psychiatric "Disorders"

From Hyperactive Kids to Anxiety and Insomnia

Actually no less than the entire world is the proper catchment area for present-day psychiatry, and psychiatry need not be alarmed by the magnitude of the task.
—Dr. H. P. Rome, past president of the American Psychiatric Association, *American Journal of Psychiatry*, 1968.

Bettelheim threatened us often with getting well or not. It was a perfect way to control us, because it left the decision entirely in his hands. Since he had decided we were crazy, he would also decide when we were well. Until then, we were at his mercy.
—Roberta C. Redford, *New York Times*, November 20, 1990, A20.

Mike Moncrief, chairman of the Texas Senate Interim Committee on Health and Human Services, tells the story of an adolescent boy who was apprehended at his grandparent's home in San Antonio by employees of a private security firm. The employees, who were not police officers, nevertheless flashed large police badges, and took the young man to a hospital where he was admitted for substance abuse problems without ever being examined by a physician or even given a drug test until four days after his admission (the test turned out to be negative). The boy was not released until a state senator intervened and a judge's order was obtained. Mr. Moncrief later found that the private security firm was being paid between $150 to $450 for each patient delivered to certain private psychiatric hospitals in the area.

His investigations also disclosed more subtle ways to fill the psychiatric hospitals. One particular corporate chain of psychiatric hospitals were promoting "Books as Hooks"—inexpensive printed materials used a marketing tools to fill a hospital's beds. "We've been suing these books for three years . . . families love these books and they do help us fill the hospital," wrote a substance abuse director.

Once the patient—or the patient's parents—had been "hooked" it wasn't so easy to get out of the hospital. As Mr. Moncrief testified at the hearings held in spring of 1992, "time and time again, throughout almost 80 hours of public testimony, witnesses gave accounts of how they were cured miraculously on the day their insurance benefits ran out—28 days seemed to be the magic number. Others related horrifying experiences of having voluntarily sought treatment for such conditions as an eating disorder or chronic back pain and then found themselves being held against their will. Still others told of having their diagnosis falsified by hospital personnel so it would match their insurance benefits."

The insurance industry, said Mr. Moncrief, failed to monitor this fraud, and one possible explanation, reported in the *Houston Chronicle*, "is that several major health insurance companies own large quantities of stock in the corporations that, in turn, own private psychiatric and other health care facilities."

In the spring of 1992, U.S. Representative Patricia Schroeder of Colorado held hearings on such practices of private psychiatric hospitals. "Our investigation has found," she said, "that thousands of adolescents, children, and adults have been hospitalized for psychiatric treatment they didn't need; that hospitals hire bounty hunters to kidnap patients with mental health insurance; that patients are kept against their will until their insurance benefits run out; that psychiatrists are being pressured by the hospitals to increase profit; that hospitals 'infiltrate' schools by paying kickbacks to school counselors who deliver students; that bonuses are paid to hospital employees, including psychiatrists, for keeping the hospital beds filled; and that military dependents are being targeted for their generous mental health benefits. I could go on, but you get the picture."

The diagnosis of psychiatric ailments has always been troublingly murky, open to varying interpretations, and can have particularly sinister consequences. While a diagnosis of any kind can work against someone, only in the case of a psychiatric diagnosis can people be forcibly detained against their will. In New York, for example, people declared incompetent by a psychiatrist—often after a brief interview—can have their rights taken away and their property seized.

As in other areas of diagnosis, there is often a very thin line between what is "diseased" and what is "normal"; feeding these diagnostic flames is the tendency of psychiatrists to take what are essentially normal problems of life and give them important-sounding names, such as "late luteal phase disorder" (premenstrual syndrome), "anxiety state," and "borderline state."

In fact, when you ask different psychiatrists to diagnose the same people, they frequently disagree, often quite wildly. In a pilot study for psychiatric insurance published in the 1960s, for example, the investigators found that while psychiatrists tended to hold to the same diagnosis *they* had made for a given patient, as soon as that patient visited another psychiatrist, the initial diagnosis was usually changed or modified. Of 73 patients who saw two different psychiatrists, only 15 were given identical diagnoses by both psychiatrists, and in 31 of the 73 where two doctors both gave their diagnoses, there was a major change. In 20 of the patients, the psychiatrists disagreed as to whether they were even dealing with a psychosis or not.

More recently, a study at a New York hospital showed that of 89 patients diagnosed with schizophrenia, only 16 actually had the disorder according to stricter diagnostic criteria. Psychiatrists Drs. Alan A. Lipton and Franklin S. Simon wrote: "The self-fulfilling prognostic prophecy of gloom in schizophrenia . . . was painfully evident in the histories of most of our patients. Most often, once written, the diagnosis of schizophrenia became irrevocable and apparently was never reconsidered." The drugs prescribed for schizophrenia, they wrote, made such reconsideration unlikely, since they were given in doses high enough to "quiet" the "disturbing" symptoms. The drugs used to treat schizophrenia cause, among other complications, tardive dyskinesia, a neuromuscular disorder similar to Parkinson's disease. These often irreversible disorders are "a terrible complication by any standard but are especially so when the drug is used inappropriately and when it is administered to patients who do not have schizophrenia," they wrote.

Robert Spitzer, M.D., the psychiatrist who headed the group that formulated the American Psychiatric Association's current diagnostic manual, stated that when researchers conduct studies of psychiatric populations, they ignore the diagnoses given by practicing psychiatrists on the assumption that they may not be accurate.

While research psychiatrists may fault the clinical diagnoses, others point to the fact that the psychiatric diagnostic manual itself may not be the bible some would hold it to be. In their view, as noted by E. Havi Morreim in the *Journal of Medicine and Philosophy*, the seemingly endless series of changes in the manual are not "the refinement of categories or cumulative gains common to advanced scientific fields, but signs of fundamental uncertainties about the nature and classification of mental illness, springing perhaps from the lack of a formal, universally accepted general theory of human thought and behavior." The late Dr. Karl Menninger, who, from the family clinic in Topeka, Kansas, helped to change how the public views mental illness, "was always skeptical about psychiatric diagnoses, and felt that doctors should study each person individually," said Dr. Alan Miller, a psychiatrist at the State University of New York at Stony Brook.

Given the chance, psychiatrists may see disease in everyone. When Robert Shepherd, M.D., compiled the case records of 1,000 patients who came to the emergency department of a large downtown teaching hospital in Montreal, and who were seen by someone from the psychiatry department, he found that 98 percent were given a psychiatric diagnosis and referred for some type of psychiatric follow-up care. Dr. Shepherd said:

But even a quick look at the records, Dr. Shepherd found, showed that the people so diagnosed were going through situations such as adolescent rebellion, marital and job problems,

excessive drinking, boredom, and loneliness. "They had problems, but did they have psychiatric illness? Yet, here they were
being labeled 'anxiety state,' 'neurotic,' 'psychotic,' 'borderline
state,' 'character disorder,' or whatever, and plugged into the
psychiatric system.

"Nobody seemed to be standing back and saying hey, wait a
minute, these people are not sick!" When the resident who
initially made the diagnosis would present the cases at rounds,
his or her superior rarely demanded evidence to support the
diagnosis. "In psychiatry you could more or less pick any label
you thought suitable, and have it validated by the clinician on
duty next day." And, once made, wrote Dr. Shepherd, the diagnoses stuck, often for months or years, and often resulting in
considerable problems for the patient so labeled.

Psychiatrist Thomas Szasz, M.D., of Syracuse, New York, has
argued that all mental illnesses not associated with lesions are
"myths." While I agree with his analysis in many respects, I don't
hold that an identifiable lesion separates disease from nondisease,
since, as we have seen, many people have lesions—fibroid tumors,
gallstones, lumpy breasts—that are totally irrelevant to their
ability to function quite normally. I have also seen people whose
psychiatric state was such that they weren't functioning normally
and represented a potential danger to themselves or others, even
though they probably had no identifiable lesions. So I will hold
to the same definition of disease stated in earlier chapters: it
becomes worthwhile to make the diagnosis of "disease" at that
stage when the benefits of diagnosis and treatment exceed the
risks. In the case of psychiatric disease, of course, the risks and
benefits to the society at large may assume a greater importance
than they do for most nonpsychiatric diseases.

THE GROWTH OF PRIVATE PSYCHIATRIC HOSPITALS

Perhaps even more than in general health care, in the mental
health field the last few years have seen a huge split in care
between those with health insurance and those without it. Formerly, most psychiatric care was paid for by the state, while
private care remained the luxury of the few who were rich enough
to pay for it. But with the "deinstitutionalization" of many of the

mentally ill, those without insurance have literally found themselves on the streets, while those people whose insurance covers mental health find themselves very much in demand as patients. The reason has been the explosive growth in the number of for-profit psychiatric hospitals, coupled with the fact that many states now require health insurance to include coverage for mental health. The number of beds in for-profit psychiatric hospitals in the United States grew from 21,400 in 1984 to 37,500 in 1990. The rate of growth was particularly large in Palm Beach County, Florida, where the number of freestanding private psychiatric hospitals grew from one to seven, while other general care hospitals also opened up psychiatric and drug and alcohol units.

As Morreim wrote in the *Journal of Medicine and Philosophy*, "As the number of inpatient beds rises to greet their newfound insurance coverage, commensurate pressures arise to find lots of mentally ill people to fill them. Psychiatry therefore is encouraged to expand the number and scope of mental illness diagnoses. . . Pressures to expand diagnostic categories translate . . . into pressure to ascribe diagnoses of mental disorder to as many patients as possible, and to hospitalize as many of these as possible. Of particular interest are pressures to label as 'disordered' persons who formerly were regarded only as obnoxious, irritable, or weak-willed."

Morreim noted that the problems are particularly marked in the case of children and adolescents. The three principal diagnoses under which they are hospitalized, he says, are (1) conduct disorders, (2) personality or childhood disorders, and (3) transitional disorders. "Conduct disorders, diagnosed on the basis of a six month pattern of such behaviors as truancy, running away from home, stealing, and persistent lying, are virtually identical to the sorts of behavior that, under other circumstances, might warrant the child's being processed through the juvenile justice system as a status offender." Here, of course, it might be argued that the child benefits from the diagnosis, since psychiatric hospitalization might be preferable to jail.

More troubling is the concept of "personality disorders," which include the sorts of stubbornness, argumentativeness, and identity crises that many developmental psychologists generally consider to be normal tensions and stages of growing up. The child may violate minor rules, throw temper tantrums, or suffer serious distress as he or she tries to resolve identity issues such as career choice, friendship patterns, or long-term personal goals. Transitional disorders are characterized by "overreaction" to identifiable stressors, such as a divorce between parents, and are acknowledged to be transitory in the great majority of cases. "Only rarely do juveniles with these diagnoses have the severity of mental illness that would be required for hospitalization of an adult," Morreim wrote.

"Most kids look psychotic at various times in their life," Walter E. Afield, M.D., a psychiatrist with the Mental Health Programs Corporation, testified at Pat Schroeder's hearings. "If they walk into a psychiatric hospital, they are going to be admitted and kept for a long period of time. . . . Because of such hospitalization, they will be prevented from getting state employment, federal employment, running for public office. Such a diagnosis," he went on, "eliminates their ability to get future medical insurance and labels them with a diagnosis forever."

HYPERACTIVITY

While hospitalization of children for supposed psychiatric disorders may be a particularly strong treatment, prescribing drugs for diagnoses such as hyperactivity (now known as attention deficit disorder) is also an area of abuse. Gunnar B. Stickler, M.D., professor emeritus of pediatrics at the Mayo Clinic, believes the diagnosis is made at least ten times, and perhaps as much as 100 times, as often as it should be.

This diagnosis, he says, is a very muddy area, as there is no particular definition as to what hyperactive means. According to an article in the *Lahey Clinic Health Letter*, which claims that attention deficit disorder (ADD) affects an estimated 2 to 10 percent of all school-age children, "Because many ADD symptoms—including impulsiveness, inattentiveness, and excessive motor activity—closely resemble what for some youngsters is normal childhood rambunctiousness, disagreement has erupted over just what constitutes a diagnosis of ADD." Dr. Stickler occasionally made the diagnosis himself, using this definition: if you have a child in your office for a few minutes and the papers get strewn all over the place, that child is hyperactive. While there are children who indeed have an attention deficit disorder, many "hyperactive" children, he believes, are simply children raised without adequate discipline.

Children who seem to be hyperactive may actually have an advantage in later life. Dr. Martin Wolfish, chief of the department of pediatrics at North York General Hospital in Willowdale, Ontario, points out that "the successful used-car dealers, the insurance salesmen, the dynamic stockbrokers of the world may well have their roots in people with the attention deficit disorder."

While in some countries, such as Britain, stimulant drugs are rarely or never used in treating ADD, one study found that in the United States in Baltimore County, Maryland, nearly six percent of *all* children were receiving stimulants to treat their ADD. Such drugs are, of course, not free of side effects.

ANXIETY, DEPRESSION, PANIC ATTACKS, AND SLEEP DISORDERS

At least once a week, it seems, a press release comes in my mail about either anxiety, depression, panic attacks, or sleep disorders. I group the four because all are related: anxious people tend to be depressed and to suffer panic attacks and sleep disorders. At least this is what the press releases tell me.

As Martha Weiman Lear wrote in the *New York Times Magazine*, all the current interest in anxiety disorders, as manifested in seminars, press releases, and articles, "is not necessarily because there is more anxiety around," but because "researchers tend to gravitate toward research dollars, and anxiety research is very popular among pharmaceutical houses that sell tranquilizers. In one day, in Montreal, three of them sponsored three different symposiums on panic attacks."

Some people with severe anxiety undoubtedly benefit from treatment. But anxiety is one of those emotions from which we all suffer now and then in some degree, and it helps us cope with our lives. Anxiety about an exam, for example, may cause us to study for it, getting a better grade. One way to handle anxiety, keeping it within the normal range of reactions, is to maintain a sense of control. As David Mechanic wrote a number a years ago,

"The awareness that one is able to cope and that one has had success in the past in dealing with adversity insulates the person from anxiety."

But because anxiety is one of those symptoms that we all have in some degree, it's easy to have a "medical students' syndrome" when we hear about this "disease." When reading about symptoms of panic attacks, who among us doesn't think back to, say, an overcrowded department store during the Christmas rush, where the air is almost unbreathable because of the mélange of perfumes that no self-respecting woman would wear singly, let alone all together? Was the perhaps desperate urge to get out a rational response to the understandable need for fresh air, or was it instead a symptom of a disease that needs a doctor's attention and probably prescription? Thinking of the experience as a need for fresh air and leaving the department store in order to get some as a rational response gives us a sense of control; thinking about the experience as a disease that needs treatment, perhaps tranquilizers, can only add to the sense that our lives are out of control. And what happens if we forgot to bring our tranquilizers?

Publicity about panic attacks often emphasizes the element of lack of control. Ian Robertson, writing in the *British Medical Journal*, described a British TV program about panic attacks that included such "mood effects," as Dr. Who-like sound, sepia monochrome film, leafless trees, and suburban trains, supposedly to convey the sense of what it's like to suffer a panic attack.

But the program did not include the role that hyperventilation plays in panic disorders, Robertson wrote, nor did anyone point out that most people who suffer panic attacks get over it themselves. The program did not explain that alarming thoughts cause panic, that panic causes changes in breathing, that changes in breathing cause physiologic changes in the body, and that physiologic changes in the body cause more panic.

"The cornerstone of panic attacks is the sufferer's perception that he or she cannot control them. The belief becomes self-perpetuating, and a vicious circle develops."

Promoting drugs for panic attacks and anxiety, rather than explaining how they occur and how they can be thwarted, is a two-edged sword. Drugs may help, at least temporarily. But as "Feeling Fit in Indiana" wrote to newspaper columnist Ann

Landers: "I became addicted to tranquilizers and tried every antidepressant on the market. Nothing worked. In fact, the drugs produced deeper feelings of anxiety and insecurity. What turned my life around was meditating, going to support group meetings, and reading books in the library on anxiety and phobias."

The author William Styron has outlined the role he believes the sleeping medication Halcion played in his suicidal thoughts during a major depression. While he doesn't claim Halcion was solely responsible for the depression, he does believe that it worsened it. "The benzodiazepines—Valium, Xanax, Ativan, and especially Halcion—are not just any drugs. Despite their occasional beneficial effects, the danger they represent should cause them to be used sparingly and given stern respect. Great progress is being made in treating depression. But unless both patient and doctor become capable of overseeing meticulously the use of these drugs, there will continue to be setbacks and, more important, losses that are mortal and beyond recovery."

Halcion is used to treat insomnia, another disorder that is poorly defined. Wang Associates, a public relations firm in health and high technology, concludes that more than 50 million Americans suffer from at least one bout of insomnia each year; symptoms include difficulty falling asleep, frequent awakenings during the night, and final awakening early in the morning. Without really noting that such short-term insomnia is probably not much of a problem for most of us (another release from a pharmaceutical public relations firm promotes insomnia as a deadly disease—"just ask any airline pilot"), the release gets to the point: a new medication for short-term insomnia has just been approved by the FDA. And *News* from the Johns Hopkins Medical Institutions tells us, "That lazy 'let me stay in bed' feeling many people have may be part of a sleep disorder" and says it is characterized by sleeping late on weekends!

What the disease-mongers don't tell us is that attempting to deal with our insomnia with drugs can sometimes cause more problems that it solves. Halcion, for example, probably poses fewer problems for the essentially healthy person taking it to treat minor insomnia or jet lag than it does for the person whose sleeplessness is a sign of serious depression. But even here the taker may find that he or she is simply trading insomnia for amnesia, or insomnia now for insomnia later. Dr. Anthony Kales, of the Pennsylvania State University College of Medicine, found that 40 percent of people taking Halcion had next-day memory impairment or amnesia. Defenders of Halcion base their case not on the fact that it doesn't impair memory, but on the fact that all benzodiazepines—the minor tranquilizers often used for insomnia—*also* impair memory.

Mark S. Silverman, M.D., of Mercy Hospital of Pittsburgh, found that the side effects of triazolam (the generic name for Halcion) are not limited to the frail elderly. One Sunday afternoon, he wrote in a letter to the *New England Journal of Medicine*, he found himself sitting at his parents' home at one in the afternoon with no memory of how he had gotten there, and indeed no memory of anything that had happened since he had gone to bed the night before in his own home three miles away. Dr. Silverman pointed out that he was a 30-year-old healthy nonsmoker, not taking any medications, and he had not been drinking.

That evening, he noticed some samples of triazolam on his bedside table and remembered that he had had insomnia, and that around 2 A.M. he had taken a 0.125 milligram tablet.

The whole experience was quite frightening, he wrote. "Needless to say, I have since avoided benzodiazepines."

Sleeping potions have been around for a long time, as anyone who's ever read *A Midsummer Night's Dream* or *Snow White* knows. In literature from ancient times, it was usually someone else who administered the sleeping potion in order to pull the wool over someone's eyes. But the pharmaceutical industry has convinced people that occasional insomnia is a medical emergency, whose risks are greater than the memory problems caused by the pills it markets to cure it. The wool is still being pulled over our eyes, but now it's *before* we take the sleeping potions rather than after.

Chapter 17

Diagnosing Our Genes

Jack: Oh, before the end of the week I shall have got rid of him. I'll say he died in Paris of apoplexy. Lots of people die of apoplexy, quite suddenly, don't they?
Algernon: Yes, but it's hereditary, my dear fellow. It's the sort of thing that runs in families. You had much better say a severe chill.
  —Oscar Wilde, *The Importance of Being Earnest*, first produced 1895.

Paul Billings, M.D., chief of genetic medicine at California-Presbyterian Medical Center, collects anecdotes about people who run into trouble because of a genetic diagnosis—or because of even the *possibility* of a genetic diagnosis. One woman, for example, who had a relative with cystic fibrosis inquired at a clinic in her small midwestern town about a test that might determine whether she was a carrier for the cystic fibrosis gene. Since she was not married—and in order to have a child with cystic fibrosis both she and her husband would have to be carriers of the gene—she decided not to pursue the matter. But when she later married, the clinic, which provided medical care for her husband's employer, *demanded* that both she and her husband have the test before they would include them in the company health plan.

If such things happen when people only *inquire* about a test, imagine what will happen to people who take a genetic test that shows that they are carriers of a gene likely to cause them problems later in life or perhaps to result in the birth of a child with a disease that insurers consider expensive.

"The consequences of such labeling, given the current situation concerning health insurance, are dismal," says Dr. Billings.

In the past, most genetic diagnoses were made by analyzing an individual's family history, for example, by creating a chart of relatives with a given disease known to be transmitted genetically, and the individual's risk was determined, sometimes relatively accurately, from such a chart. More recently, tests have been developed in which the chromosomes themselves are examined for the presence of genes that transmit disease. Such tests can predict a proportion of cases of cystic fibrosis, find a gene (called p53) associated with breast and colon cancer, and detect a chromosome (the fragile X) discovered in association with mental retardation.

The recent discovery that defective genes may expand as they pass from parent to child, resulting in more severe genetic disease in each generation, adds a new wrinkle to the issue. It now may be possible to detect genetic defects that are unlikely to be serious to the person in whom they are detected—but which may indicate serious disease several generations down the line.

Commercial and other labs are now offering a variety of genetic tests, and press articles almost daily hail the advances in genetics, only sometimes adding the caveat that such tests might be used against individuals for insurance purposes. A press release announcing GeneScreen, Inc., the first genetic screening laboratory in the north Texas area, noted that it was offering a test for susceptibility to insulin-dependent or Type I diabetes.

What's interesting here is that there's already a nongenetic test that can predict susceptibility to both Type I and Type II diabetes, known as the glucose tolerance test. Many diabetologists, however, do not recommend having such a test because knowing you are susceptible to diabetes does little good and can cause considerable harm. "The most important thing you could do for your readers," says F. John Service, M.D., Ph.D., a professor of medicine and diabetologist at the Mayo Clinic, "is to discourage them from having a glucose tolerance test." The diagnosis sometimes made by this test is impaired glucose tolerance, a risk factor for diabetes. "We don't make that diagnosis here," says Dr. Service, "probably because of perceived insurance problems." A genetic test for susceptibility to Type I diabetes may even be less useful than the glucose tolerance test, since the glucose tolerance test also predicts susceptibility to Type II diabetes, and you can reduce your risk of developing Type II diabetes by keeping your weight under control. But there's no way, at least at present, to reduce your risk of Type I diabetes, calling into question the need for such a test.

Michael Kaback, M.D., chairman of pediatrics at the University of California at San Diego, cautions that the test for the cystic fibrosis gene is likely to do more harm than good, particularly if widely used. "But people get caught up in this simplistic view that the test will prevent disease and get on a fast track to deliver it." He feels that the test should be offered only to people who have cystic fibrosis in their families. For one thing, he says, the test will have a higher predictive value in these people. For another, they know what having a child with cystic fibrosis means in terms of daily life, and they are in a much better position to judge the consequences than are other people, who may believe the condition is worse than it really is.

As we have seen in the case of other tests, genetic tests are often promoted without anybody's really understanding what they *mean*. "As a medical geneticist, I know more than the average physician," says Dr. Billings. "Yet I don't know how to interpret a finding that the p53 gene [a gene found in many breast and colon cancers] is present, and I'm not sure what finding the fragile X means in an individual not noticeably retarded."

If medical geneticists don't know how to interpret genetic information, imagine what the quality of information given out by the average physician is—and what the consequences can be. One man, for example, with a family history of Charcot-Marie-Tooth (CMT) disease, a genetic disease that causes progressive atrophy of the muscles, was instructed by his physician "never to have any children," even though he showed no symptoms of the disease. The physician apparently didn't understand that CMT disease is inherited as a dominant gene, which means that while the patient had a 50 percent chance of having the disease, if he didn't have the disease himself, he wouldn't pass it on to his children. Since the signs of this disease appear fairly early in life, as each succeeding year went by without symptoms, his chances of being affected decreased. "By age 27 years, persons at risk but with no clinical manifestations have less than a 3 percent chance of having inherited the gene, and by age 35 years the chance is essentially zero," wrote Kathryn H. Spitzer and Dr. Lytt I. Gardner in the *Journal of the American Medical Association*. No one had ever told the man this, however. When he was 35, he and his wife had a child, and two years later he sought genetic counseling due to the guilt and fear that he had passed a debilitating disease on to his child. "He described his fear that he would eventually contract the disease himself almost as a concrete object—a lump in his consciousness every day of his life."

The news that there was virtually no risk that he inherited the gene and was unlikely to pass it to his descendants, "was like a reprieve to a condemned man. It was as though the specter of a dread disease had been exorcised from him."

BRIGHT SPOTS

In many ways the use of genetic tests is no different from the use of other medical tests, particularly those for risk factors such as high cholesterol, since both types of test are used not to see why an individual is sick, but to predict what may happen to him or her in the future. But there are two bright spots in the use of genetic tests that aren't found concerning most other medical tests. One is that a group of dedicated geneticists has kept the issue of the hazards of "genetic screening" in the public eye, and there are genetic counselors around the country trained in educating people to evaluate correctly the risks and consequences of genetic testing.

The other bright spot is that while insurance companies will use the information from any screening tests that a person has voluntarily undergone, they currently are not screening people for genetic diseases themselves. That's partly because it's expensive—a test for Huntington's disease can cost several thousand dollars—and partly because they realize that genetic screening might open a Pandora's box that could ultimately bring down the insurance industry. After all, genetic screening might determine that *everybody* is at risk for disease, undermining the whole concept of risk rating. If everybody were to be excluded from coverage, there would be no one to pay premiums and no insurance industry. As an article in *Medical World News* pointed out, almost all assembled experts at a recent conference agreed that the impact of genetic testing on insurability will help push the United States toward some type of universal health care access program.

While so far no insurance companies seem to be requiring genetic testing, they will use any information they can get if a patient has had a genetic test for other reasons, and they almost certainly won't use it in a way that serves the patient's interest. A major conclusion of the genetic testing committee of the American Council of Life Insurance is that insurers must avoid applicants who undergo genetic testing and withhold the results, so this information appearing almost anywhere on your medical records would be potentially dangerous. "Almost every insurer in the business would immediately revise an applicant's risk rating when presented with genetic test results," Robert Pokorski, medical director of Lincoln National Life Insurance Company, Fort Wayne, Indiana, told *Medical World News*. The same is true for a family history that may suggest an increased risk of genetically transmitted disease.

Nancy Wexler, Ph.D., president of the Hereditary Disease Foundation at Columbia University, tells the story of a woman in Michigan who had two siblings affected by colon cancer. In order to try to detect whether she, too, had the disease, she underwent an examination of the colon known as a colonosocopy, which showed that her colon was perfectly normal.

When she later applied for a health insurance policy, she found it contained a rider excluding all coverage of procedures relating to her colon, even though neither she nor any of her physicians discussed the family history of colon cancer with the insurance company.

As Dr. Wexler told the U.S. House of Representatives on October 17, 1991, "If she should develop colon cancer in the future, she would have to assume all treatment costs herself—an impossibility. She cannot even afford to pay for the colonoscopies that might minimize the cost of any cancer through early detection."

Just why the insurance company decided to deny this woman insurance for her colon—whether it decided that anyone who has a colonoscopy is suspect, whether the history was mentioned on the form requisitioning the examination, or whether the insurance company found something in a previous medical record about the history of colon cancer—will remain a mystery. As David A. Testone pointed out, based on his experience with the Special Services (S.S.) unit of Mutual of Omaha, it's not called the S.S. for nothing.

This is not to say that you should *never* get a genetic test. Couples who want to find out whether they will have a deformed child, for example, may feel that whatever the risks of being labeled, they are worth not giving birth to a child with a serious deformity. Finding that you are at risk for a serious disease may be worthwhile if in fact there are measures you can take to avoid that disease—and if you'll be able to afford those measures if you can't get health insurance. If you know from your family history that you're at risk for a serious hereditary disease, a genetic test may give you a reprieve by showing that you have not, indeed, inherited the gene(s) in question.

But don't submit to a genetic test without giving serious thought to all the consequences, medical, social, psychological, and financial. Find a doctor or genetic counselor who can help guide you through this. Find out whether you can do anything to prevent development of the disease and whether these measures might just as well be taken without the genetic tests. Make sure your insurance is in order—insofar as possible—*before* you have the test. Dr. Reed Pyeritz, clinical director of the Johns Hopkins Center for Medical Genetics in Baltimore, for example, advises his patients that, "rather than trying to purchase a $250,000 life insurance policy, they buy ten $25,000 policies, which don't get scrutinized as closely."

Getting a health insurance house in order isn't easy in today's economy of layoffs and bankruptcies, since insurance that comes with the job is usually lost with the job, and many health insurance plans are going bankrupt. A genetic diagnosis is for life, so you must hope your health insurance holds up that long, or at least until you become old enough for Medicare or poor enough for Medicaid.

Chapter 18

Putting Disease in Its Place

A Prescription for Change

Knock: In 250 of the houses you see . . . there are 250 rooms where someone confesses to medicine, 250 beds where a body witnesses that life has meaning, and thanks to me a medical meaning. At night it's even more beautiful because there are lights. And almost all the light belongs to me: those who aren't sick sleep in darkness, they're not important.

    Think about it, that everybody's first duty is to remember my prescription.

    Think about it: in a few minutes the clock will strike ten, which is the time when everybody takes their rectal temperature for the second time. In a few minutes 250 thermometers will penetrate at the same time.

    —Jules Romains, *Knock.*

Health economist Uwe Reinhardt paints a vivid verbal picture to illustrate the direction that medical care is going in the United States. Imagine, says Reinhardt, two people on a bed with tubes running alongside bringing them nourishment from abroad. He then explains that America is currently putting over 12 percent of our gross national product (GNP) into health care, up from 9 percent in 1980. At this rate we'll be spending a third of all our resources on medicine within 20 years, and if the proportion continues to rise, some day 100 percent of the GNP will be taken up by health care, which means that all Americans will be able to do is to lie on beds administering medical care to each other, with everything else we need, like food and water, produced abroad and transported to us via the tubes.

Americans have been seduced by the idea that greater competition in health care would reduce costs and improve services as doctors, drug companies, and insurance companies competed with one another for health care dollars. Instead, competition in American health care has developed into a two-headed monster, one head creating diseases and the other discarding patients.

Competition in medical care has failed either to contain prices or to provide adequate service, because within the current system health care providers and drug companies are prompted to increase the demand for medical services indefinitely by defining more and more people—as long as they have insurance—as sicker and sicker. Competition among the insurers is based not on providing superior services, but on weeding out "bad risks," or even those simply perceived as being "bad risks." People "diagnosed" on the basis of the competition among providers may then become uninsurable based on the competition among the payers.

What can be done?

One possible solution would be a system of national health insurance in which payment for doctors was based not on diagnoses, nor on items of service, but on either salary or "capitation," the number of people on a given doctor's list. Such a scheme would cut down on disease mongering in two important ways.

First, it would help distribute the nation's doctors over the entire population. The current maldistribution was poignantly illustrated by two stories juxtaposed on the same page of a recent *Newsday*. On the left-hand side was a story about long waits at one of New York City's public hospitals, and on the right was a story about how one of the city's private hospitals was offering bounties to ambulance drivers for every insured patient they could bring to that hospital. Too many doctors are chasing after the portion of the population that has health insurance, which also tends to be that portion of the population that is already healthier, since these people couldn't get insurance if they weren't healthy. A uniform system of payment would make it as profitable to treat a truly sick patient as to convince a well one that he or she is sick, and it's probably a lot more satisfying, too.

Second, a payment system based on salary and capitation would eliminate incentives for overdiagnosis and overtreatment. Unfortunately, it might also tend to make doctors lazy, since they would be paid the same no matter how much they worked. This, to some extent, has happened in England under the National Health Service, but it may be the lesser of the evils: English people have life expectancies comparable to those for Americans, and they achieve it at much less cost.

While a system of national health insurance that didn't reward overdiagnosis or overtreatment would probably be the best solution to disease mongering, partial measures might help if they were intelligently designed. Perhaps competition could be made to work better, but doing so would mean regulating the terms upon which providers and insurers compete.

We the public should insist that health care providers compete, not on the basis of the number of glitzy machines that mostly serve to convince us we are ill when we're not, but on the basis of superior service using an honest appraisal of the risks and benefits of diagnosis and treatment. We should choose not the doctor who orders the most tests, but the one who does the best job explaining what the ordered tests *mean*. We should also insist that insurers compete on the basis of service, not on the basis of refusing to insure people with either real or perceived health problems. We can't expect them to do this on their own: laws outlawing risk rating by insurance companies will be necessary. As Nancy Kass, of the program in Law, Ethics, and Health of the Johns Hopkins School of Hygiene and Public Health, has written, "Precedent exists for insurance companies to classify applicants by risk and to make exclusions accordingly. However, precedent also exists for insurers and, certainly, for other private businesses, to be regulated when there are overriding social or public policy concerns."

An alternative way to abolish the practice of risk rating would be to institute much stricter legislation regarding medical privacy. Currently, all health insurers send information to a central data bank in Massachusetts, so any time one insurer obtains information, all insurers have access to it. While there are federal privacy laws, they apply only to the government. There is no national forum for people to take complaints when they feel their privacy has been invaded by businesses. Making it a crime, or at least more difficult, to disclose medical records would make risk rating much more difficult and perhaps ultimately unrewarding.

CAVEAT EMPTOR

Finally, until some sort of policy is instituted with regard to risk rating, every person who has to buy individual policies of health insurance should be a savvy buyer. If you have a preexisting condition that you do not want to admit to, make certain that there is no way the insurance company can find out about it, either through your medical records, your pharmacy, or facts on file about you at the central data bank in Massachusetts. (To find out just what your file says, you can write the Medical Information Bureau, P.O. Box 105, Essex Station, Boston, MA 02112, or call them at 617-426-3660.)

If you are currently applying for an individual policy and are telling your doctor to release your medical records, sit down together and find out exactly what's on them. If the doctor has written something such as "Rule out gastritis," you may be denied insurance even if you were subsequently found not to have gastritis. David A. Testone, an insurance consultant in Brewster, New York, says that insurance companies look for the diagnosis, the frequency of treatment, the type of treatment, and the prognosis (but as we saw in chapter 1, most cannot recognize the diagnosis of a nonexistent disease). Be certain that what you put on your medical questionnaire is in accord with what's on your records. Even failing to mention a common and—among women—almost ubiquitous symptom such as vaginitis can allow an insurance company to cancel your policy because it claims that you lied about a preexisting condition. Testone cites the case of a man who had a heart attack, and a check of his medical records found that he had been advised to go on a low-fat, low-cholesterol diet. The company bought back his policy, meaning that he was left without insurance, but now with an important preexisting condition. The preexisting condition doesn't have to be related to the one you may be making a claim for. "If they find anything at all they'll use it—it doesn't have to be related."

An important notion to keep in mind is that insurance policies have a contestable period, usually lasting from 11 months to 2 years, and usually noted in fine print on the last page. If you file a claim during the contestable period, explains Testone, it's almost certain to be challenged: "They'll contest any claim in the contestable period." Anything on your medical record that you didn't mention can be taken as evidence that you lied. Once you have held the policy for the contestable period, it's much less likely to be questioned. So when possible, avoid making claims during the contestable period. You should also choose a company that's not likely to go bankrupt and, if possible, stay with that company. Switching to another might result in somewhat lower rates, but it also means that you may not have coverage when you need it.

DEALING WITH DR. KNOCKS

An informed consumer is probably the best defense against Knock-like physicians who try to convince well patients that they are really sick. Better use can and should be made of second opinions; for example, under current procedures insurers often require a patient to seek a second opinion for surgery from a surgical specialist. It would make more sense to get the second opinion from someone who normally treated the disease in question without surgery. For example, if removal of an endocrine gland is recommended, the second opinion should come from a medical endocrinologist. If a hysterectomy is recommended on the basis that fibroid tumors pose a threat to the kidneys, a condition that gynecologists seem to believe is common but other doctors— including those specializing in kidney disease—believe rare, it makes more sense to have a nephrologist, or kidney specialist, rather than another gynecologist, rule on the need for surgery.

Some people would suggest that doctors be prohibited from referring patients to themselves for costly procedures. A cardiologist, for example, would not be allowed to perform angiography, but should instead refer a patient to someone else, for example, an interventional radiologist. Such mandatory referrals could help ensure that the procedure is recommended for the good of the patient, not of the doctor's pocketbook. While some sort of prohibition might be built into insurance schemes, you can, to some extent, protect yourself from overdiagnosis and over-treatment by chosing a family practitioner or general internist to consult before any medical procedure. If the family practitioner wants you to have an X-ray procedure such as a mammogram, insist on referral to a radiologist skilled in interpreting this test.

The most intelligent use of health resources depends upon a strong system of primary care physicians such as family practitioners and general internists, who are trained in the importance of talking to patients, and in performing or prescribing tests and procedures only when the consequences of such tests are fully considered. Unfortunately, physicians are paid better for doing tests than for talking and using good judgment, and until the reimbursement scheme changes significantly, there will be significant incentives for overtesting.

QUI TAM

In blatant cases of "Knockism," perhaps more use ought to be made of the legal principle of *qui tam*. (The name comes from the Latin: *Qui tam pro domino rege quam pro se ipso in hac parte sequitur* and means "one who sues on behalf of the king as well as for himself."] This is a 1986 False Claims Act Amendment that authorizes private citizens to sue on behalf of the U.S. government to recover federal funds from fraudulent recipients such as those practicing Medicare fraud. According to the National Health Care Anti-Fraud Association, fraud may account for as much as $75 billion of health care spending each year in this country. The private citizen who sues the recipient of federal funds for making a false claim is entitled to take home a part of the proceeds. The legislation is unusual in that the private citizen doesn't have to be injured by the fraudulent practices but is acting as a whistle blower. According to Dr. David C. Hsia, writing in the *Annals of Internal Medicine*, "Fraudulent practices against which *qui tam* actions may be used include billing for noncovered services (such as experimental treatments), double billing (for example, receiving two-part reimbursement for a single radiology-anesthesiology-pathology service), providing poor quality care (such as that received in Medicaid mills), providing unnecessary services (such as extra-cranial-intracranial bypass surgery), and billing the federal payer as primary for services on which another payer is primary."

We also ought to take a closer look at who's benefiting from payment based on diagnosis-related groups. These groups were based on the fact that diseases were "things" and that everyone with the same "disease" would have similar needs for medical care. When it was realized that not all people with the same label had the same need for medical care, health economists started trying to revise the DRGs, first to relate to the severity of the condition, then to relate to patient characteristics. The DRGs are becoming more and more complicated, but are they becoming more accurate? The DRG system threatens to undermine whatever diagnostic accuracy doctors have had, as computer programs teach them how to creep, or leap, the diagnosis up into a higher reimbursement category. And there's no evidence that they have slowed the rise in health care costs.

EMPLOYMENT RIGHTS

The situation with regard to employment of the person labeled with a disease *should be* getting rosier. As of 1992, the Americans with Disabilities Act (ADA) prohibits preemployment physicals at least until a job offer has been made and will generally prohibit employers from asking any questions about health except whether a given condition will actually prevent the person from performing the job. Businesses employing more than 25 persons came under the law in January 1992, and those employing more than 15 will do so in 1994.

But Mark Rothstein, a lawyer who directs the Health Law and Policy Institute at the University of Houston, says that the law, by itself, probably won't end the issue. "Given the strong economic incentives, we have to anticipate that some employers will still be willing to use preemployment health tests."

The language of ADA led people to believe that this law would protect not only people who were actually handicapped but also those *perceived* to be handicapped, such as those labeled with risk factors or genetic diagnoses. Unfortunately, in 1992, as this book was going to press, the Equal Employment Opportunity Commission, which has the responsibility for enforcing the law, was not interpreting it this way. In other words, people in wheelchairs are protected against employment discrimination, but people who have high blood pressure may not be. The law also outlaws refusing someone employment on the basis that the new employee would raise the employer's health insurance costs. But while the law says a company cannot refuse to employ someone, it may not be able to mandate that the employee get equal health care benefits. Some 70 percent of the work force in the United States work for companies that self-insure; these policies of self-insurance are not regulated by state insurance commissioners, and employees will therefore have little recourse if the company policy excludes them, or perhaps any condition they may have.

Whether the law has any impact will depend upon how rigorously it is enforced, and the more people who complain, the better for everyone. Ellen Saideman, of New York Lawyers for the Public Interest in Manhattan, suggests that anyone given a preemployment health questionnaire should send it to a group, such as hers, interested in enforcing this law.

In terms of disease mongering by pharmaceutical firms, the more aggressive stance being taken by the FDA regarding truth in pharmaceutical advertising and in food labeling can only be praised. Probably the growth in programs for training science journalists should help here, too, creating a class of journalists who will be more immune to manipulation. But the journalists with the best training don't always get the best jobs, and improving press coverage of medicine will also mean that those who hire medical journalists must begin to see medical articles as serious journalism, not as puff pieces to draw advertisers.

Postgraduate education of physicians should ideally be paid for by money that doesn't come from pharmaceutical firms, since this tends to give the companies a say in selecting topics, speakers, and slants. This idea may seem utopian, since there's no immediate answer for where else such money might come from. One possible response could be that in order to get continuing medical education credits, which allow physicians to be recertified in their specialties, they would have to participate in a certain percentage of programs NOT sponsored by the pharmaceutical, or indeed any other, industry. Fees for such courses could be tax-deductible. Another, albeit less desirable, solution would be for pharmaceutical firms to give money for continuing education programs with no strings attached.

Given the number of well-trained, sophisticated physicians who voluntarily admitted in interviews for this book that they often didn't understand the validity of tests, even tests in their own area of expertise, there seems to be a crying need for someone without an interest in pushing tests to fill this gap in physician education. The Centers for Disease Control issues reports on the infectious diseases, the FDA reports on new drugs approved, and the *Medical Letter* reports on the use of drugs. Yet there is no easy way for physicians to find out whether the tests they are ordering have a reasonable chance of helping their patients or whether they are embarking on a diagnostic snipe hunt.

PUTTING DISEASE IN PERSPECTIVE

Finally, to cope with the psychological effect of disease labeling, we as individuals need to put disease in its place, to realize that disease labels are imprecise hypotheses developed by doctors to talk to each other, and that they often don't mean that much. We as patients will have to accept the fact that many diagnoses are simply "placebo" diagnoses given either because we demand them or because the reimbursement scheme does. We must learn to accept that we may sometimes be better off without any diagnosis at all and that medicine cannot always find a reason for our aches and pains. In no case should we allow the label to become the person. Eventually, we shall all fall prey to disease, and ultimately to death, no matter what we or our doctors do. But let's not waste the lives we have worrying so much about it.

KNOCK'S VISION

Knock's vision of everyone who counts taking his or her temperature at a given hour has been realized in today's America, although instead of taking our temperatures we talk about our cholesterol. Is Reinhardt's projection of a country with no resources for anything but medical care a vision of the future? Are the overall risks of diagnosing so many nondiseases, trivial diseases, or untreatable diseases going to exceed the benefits, as people pay for pills, surgery, and diagnostic tests rather than for schools, decent housing, cultural activities, and yes, medical care that really works for those who are truly in need of it?

Both as individuals and as a society we need to put disease in its place, recognizing its infinitely expansible definitions that, in the absence of more skepticism, threaten to engulf us both as people and as a nation. Knock would have been very happy in today's America. But are we?

Notes

CHAPTER 1. *The Disease Mongers*

1. Alasdair Breckenridge, Editorial: "Treating mild hypertension," *British Medical Journal* 291, no. 6488 (July 13, 1985): 89–90.

2. David Eddy et al., "The Value of Mammography Screening in Women Under Age 50 Years," *Journal of the American Medical Association* 259, no. 10 (March 11, 1988): 1512–19.

3. Thomas McKeown, *The Role of Medicine: Dream, Mirage or Nemesis?* (Princeton, NJ: Princeton University Press, 1979), 7.

4. G. D. Smith and J. Pekkanen, "Should There Be a Moratorium on the Use of Cholesterol-Lowering Drugs?" *British Medical Journal*, 304 (1992): 431–34.

5. Allan S. Brett, "Psychologic Effects of the Diagnosis and Treatment of Hypercholesterolemia: Lessons from Case Studies," *American Journal of Medicine* 91 (1991): 642–47.

6. College of General Practitioners, *Evidence of the College of General Practitioners to the Royal Commission on Medical Education*, Reports from General Practice Number 5 (London: The College, 1966).

7. Jules Romains, *Knock* (Paris: Editions Gallimard, 1924).

8. Dena Bunis, "Dems' Health Bill Asks Employers to 'Play or Pay,'" *Newsday*, January 23, 1992, 17.

9. Thomas B. Graboys, "Conflicts of Interest in the Management of Silent Ischemia," *Journal of the American Medical Association* 261 (April 14, 1989): 2116–17.

10. D. W. Simborg, "DRG Creep: A New Hospital-Acquired Disease," *New England Journal of Medicine* 304 (1981): 1602–04; John E. Wennberg, Klim McPherson, and Philip Caper, "Will Payment Based on Diagnosis-Related Groups Control Hospital Costs?" *New England Journal of Medicine* 311, no. 5 (August 2, 1984): 295–300.

11. Susan Horn, personal communication.

12. David A. Kessler, "Drug Promotion and Scientific Exchange: The Role of the Clinical Investigator," *New England Journal of Medicine* 325, no. 3(July 18, 1991): 201–03.

13. Carl J. Pepine et al. "ACC/AHA Guidelines for Cardiac Catheterization and Cardiac Catheterization Laboratories," *Journal of the American College of Cardiology* 18(no. 5) (November 1, 1991): 1149–82.

14. David M. Eddy, "Screening for Colorectal Cancer," *Annals of Internal Medicine* 113, no. 5 (September 1, 1990): 373–84.

15. *Annals of Surgery* 125 (1990): 1032–35.

16. "Tests for Malaria May Have Spread AIDS," *Reuters*, October 28, 1990.

17. James H. Warram et al., "Excess Mortality Associated with Diuretic Therapy in Diabetes Mellitus," *Archives of Internal Medicine* 151 (July 1991): 1350–56.

18. Michael F. Oliver, "Doubts About Preventing Coronary Heart Disease," *British Medical Journal* 304 (February 15, 1992): 393–94.

19. Benjamin P. Sachs et al., "Home Monitoring of Uterine Activity: Does It Prevent Prematurity," *New England Journal of Medicine* 325, no. 19 (November 7, 1991): 1374–77.

20. Andrea M. Tree, Letter, "Effect of Check-Ups Every Three Years," *British Medical Journal* 300 (January 13, 1990): 122.

21. Mary Ann Bailey and Philip Rosenthal, "Insurability of Pediatric Gastrointestinal Disorders," *Clinical Pediatrics* 28, no. 2 (February 1989): 60–63.

22. John Markoff, "Europe Takes the Lead in Privacy Protection," *New York Times*, April 14, 1991, E9.

23. Dorothy Thompson, "Is This the Way We Want to Go?" *British Medical Journal* 307 (March 30, 1991): 795.

24. Michael W. Miller, "Patients' Records Are Treasure Trove for Budding Industry," *Wall Street Journal*, February 27, 1992, 1.

25. Seth Mydans, "Names List Leads to Ethics Debate," *New York Times*, July 30, 1991, A10.

26. M. J. Campion et al., "Psychosexual Trauma of an Abnormal Cervical Smear," *British Journal of Obstetrics and Gynecology* 95 (January 1988): 175–81.

27. Theresa M. Marteau, "Psychological Costs of Screening," Editorial, *British Medical Journal* 299 (August 26, 1989): 527.

28. John F. Burnum, "The Worried Sick," *Annals of Internal Medicine* 88, no. 4 (April 1978) 572.

29. Sandra Blakeslee, "Study Links Emotions to Second Heart Attacks," *New York Times*, September 20, 1990, B8.

30. Simon Lovestone and Thomas Fahy, "Psychological Factors in Breast Cancer," *British Medical Journal* 302 (May 25, 1991): 1219–20.

31. Daniel Goldman, "Mortality Study Lends Weight to Patient's Opinion," *New York Times* Health, March 21, 1991, B13.

32. McKeown, *Role of Medicine*, 127.

33. Arthur J. Barsky, *Worried Sick* (Boston: Little, Brown, 1988).

CHAPTER 2. *A Disease Is Not A "Thing"*

1. Karl Kraus, "Half-Truths and One and a Half Truths," quoted in "Minerva," *British Medical Journal* 292 (April 19, 1986): 1082.

2. Michael O'Donnell, "Got a Political Hot Potato? Call It a Disease," *Medical Post*, June 25, 1985, 23.

3. Susan Love, *Dr. Susan Love's Breast Book* (Reading, Mass.: Addison-Wesley 1990).

4. Samuel Vaisrub, "The Magic of a Name," *Journal of the American Medical Association* 243, no. 19 (May 16, 1980): 1931.

5. E. J. M. Campbell, J. G. Scadding, and R. S. Roberts, "The Concept of Disease," *British Medical Journal* 2 (1979): 757–62.

6. Jerome P. Kassirer and Richard I. Kopelman, "Diagnosis by Fiat," *Hospital Practice* 25 (January 15, 1990): 31–38.

7. R. Cervera, M. A. Khamashta, and G. R. V. Hughes, "Overlap Syndromes," *Annals of Rheumatic Diseases* 49 (1990): 947–48.

8. Lynn Payer, *Medicine and Culture* (New York: Henry Holt, 1988).

9. E. H. Reynolds, "Editorial: A Single Seizure," *British Medical Journal* 297 (December 3, 1988): 1422–23.

10. Editorial, "Recurrent Brief Depression and Anxiety," *Lancet* 337 (March 9, 1991): 586–87.

11. Stanley J. Reiser, "The Clinical Record in Medicine Part 1: Learning from Cases," *Annals of Internal Medicine* 114, no. 10 (May 15, 1991): 902–07.

12. Robert M. Wachter et al., "Decision About Resuscitation: Inequities Among Patients with Different Diseases but Similar Prognoses," *Annals of Internal Medicine* 111 (1989): 525–32.

13. J. G. Scadding, "Diagnosis: The Clinician and the Computer," *Lancet* (October 21, 1967): 877–82.

14. "Computer-Assisted Diagnosis," *Lancet* (December 9, 1989): 1371.

15. Joseph D. Wassersug, "Never Shrug Off the Reason the Patient Came to See You," *Medical Economics* 67 (December 10, 1990): 97–98.

16. Jerome P. Kassirer, "Letter: Our Stubborn Quest for Diagnostic Certainty," *New England Journal of Medicine*, 321, no. 18 (Nov. 2, 1989), 1273.

17. Felicity Barringer, "Many Surgeons Reassure Their Patients on Implants," *New York Times* Living Section, January 29, 1992, C1–C12.

18. Clifton K. Meador, "The Art and Science of Nondisease," *New England Journal of Medicine* (January 14, 1965): 92–95.

19. "Summary of Discussion," *Transactions of the European Orthodontic Society* (1973): 502.

20. Olga Lechky, "Going by the Book Can Slow Diagnostic Process," *Medical Post*, October 9, 1979, 59.

21. Maja Nielsen, Jorn Jensen, and Johan Andersen, "Precancerous and Cancerous Breast Lesions During Lifetime and at Autopsy: A Study of 83 Women," *Cancer* 54 (1984): 612–15.

22. Martin Reincke et al., "The 'Incidentaloma' of the Pituitary Gland: Is Neurosurgery Required?" *Journal of the American Medical Association* 263, no. 20 (May 23/30, 1990): 2772–76.

23. I. Glambek, B. Arnesjo, and O. Soreide, "Correlation Between Gallstones and Abdominal Symptoms in a Random Population," *Scandinavian Journal of Gastroenterology* 24 (1989): 277–81.

24. Jack Ratner et al., "The Prevalence of Gallstone Disease in Very Old Institutionalized Persons," *Journal of the American Medical Association* 265, no. 7 (February 20, 1991): 902–03.

25. Roar Johnsen et al., "Prevalences of Endoscopic and Histological Findings in Subjects with and Without Dyspepsia," *British Medical Journal* 302 (March 30, 1991): 749–52.

26. D. G. Colin-Jones and P. L. Golding, "What Is a Normal Upper Gastrointestinal Tract? One That Has Been Underinvestigated?" *British Medical Journal* 302 (March 30, 1991): 742.

27. Harry Bakwin, "Pseudodoxia Pediatrica," *New England Journal of Medicine,* 232, no. 24 (June 14, 1945): 691–697.

28. Nancy G. Hildreth, Roy E. Shore, and Philip M. Dvoretsky, "The Risk of Breast Cancer After Irradiation of the Thymus in Infancy," *New England Journal of Medicine* 321, no. 19 (November 9, 1989): 1281–84.

29. Kathryn Anastos et al., "Hypertension in Women: What Is Really Known?" *Annals of Internal Medicine* 115 (1991): 287–93.

30. Harvey McConnell, "'Sick' Behaviors," *The Journal* (Addiction Research Foundation of Ontario) (January 1, 1989): 16.

31. Marlon T. Gieser, Letter, "Are You Codependent?" *New York Times Book Review*, March 18, 1990, 34.

32. Ellen Goodman, "Addict, Sure, But Kitty Is More Than That," *Newsday*, September 18, 1990, 54. Copyright 1990, The Boston Globe Newspaper Co./Washington Post Writer's Group. Reprinted with permission.

33. Thomas S. Szasz, "What Counts as Disease?" *Canadian Medical Association Journal* 135 (October 15, 1986): 859.

CHAPTER 3. *The Misuse of Diagnostic Tests*

1. "Controversy Breeds Ignorance," *British Medical Journal* 302 (April 20, 1991): 973–74; Stuart Logan and Pat Tookey, Letter, "Controversy Breeds Ignorance," *British Medical Journal* 302, (May 25, 1991): 1272.

2. Milt Freudenheim, "Debate Widens Over Expanding Use and Growing Cost of Medical Tests," *New York Times*, May 30, 1987, 49.

3. Physician Payment Review Commission, "Fee Update and Medicare Volume Performance, Standards for 1992," no. 91–93, 1991.

4. Glenn Kramon, "Good Medicine, Better Business," *New York Times*, May 15, 1988, 6.

5. "Death from Lead Exposure Prompts Call for Yearly Tests," *New York Times*, March 29, 1991, B6.

6. Catherine M. Hutchinson et al., "CD4 Lymphocyte Concentrations in Patients with Newly Identified HIV Infection Attending STD Clinics," *Journal of the American Medical Association* 266, no. 2 (July 10, 1991): 253–56.

7. Erik Eckholm, "More Than Inspiration Is Needed to Fight AIDS," *New York Times*, Week in Review, November 17, 1991, 1.

8. Robert Pear, "1988 Standards for Medical Labs Go Unenforced by Administration," *New York Times*, March 20, 1991, 1.

9. Charles Marwick and Phil Gunby, "Clinical Laboratory Improvement Amendments Finally May Go Into Effect September 1," *Journal of the American Medical Association* 267, no. 11 (March 18, 1992): 1441.

10. J. L. Gordon et al., "Human Platelet Reactivity During Stressful Diagnostic Procedures," *Journal of Clinical Pathology* 26 (1973): 958–62; Alan I. Fleischman, Marvin L. Bierenbam, and Arleane Stier, "Effect of Stress Due to Anticipated Minor Surgery Upon In Vivo Platelet Aggregation in Humans," *Journal of Human Stress* (March 1976): 33–37.

11. Peter Rasmussen, "Use of the Laboratory in Patient Management," *American Family Physician* 35, no. 2 (February 1987): 214–22.

12. Lynn Payer, *How to Avoid a Hysterectomy* (New York: Pantheon, 1987).

13. "20/20," June 9, 1989.

14. Brian Berube, "Clinical Efficacy of Lab Test May Be Acid Test of Future," *Medical Post*, October 7, 1986, 15.

15. Asa J. Wilbourn and Richard J. Lederman, Letter, "Evidence for Conduction Delay in Thoracic-Outlet Syndrome Is Challenged," *New England Journal of Medicine* 310, no. 16 (April 19, 1984): 1052–53.

16. Arnold S. Relman, "Responsibilities of Authorship: Where Does the Buck Stop?" *New England Journal of Medicine* 310, no. 16 (April 19, 1984): 1048–49.

17. Peter S. Vig, "Respiration, Nasal Airway, and Orthodontics: A Review of Current Clinical Concepts and Research," *New Vistas in Orthodontics*, Lysle E. Johnston, Ed., (Philadelphia: Lea & Febiger, 1985).

18. Christopher L. Keall and Peter S. Vig, "An Improved Technique for the Simultaneous Measurement of Nasal and Oral Respiration," *American Journal of Orthodontics and Dentofacial Orthopedics* 91, no. 3 (March 1987): 207–12.

19. Peter S. Vig, Peter M. Spalding, and Ronald R. Lints, "Sensitivity and Specificity of Diagnostic Tests for Impaired Nasal Respiration," *American Journal of Orthodontics and Dentofacial Orthopedics* 99 (1991): 354–60.

20. Steven H. Woolf and Douglas B. Kamerow, "Testing for Uncommon Conditions: The Heroic Search for Positive Test Results," *Archives of Internal Medicine* 150 (December 1990): 2451–58.

21. "Devastating Findings," *U.S. News & World Report*, November 23, 1987, 68.

22. Klemens B. Meyer and Stephen G. Pauker, "Screening for HIV: Can We Afford the False Positive Rate?" *New England Journal of Medicine* 317, no. 4 (July 23, 1988): 238–41.

23. David Morgan, "AIDS Stigma in Insurance Market," *British Medical Journal* 299 (December 16, 1989): 1536.

24. Richard Wernick, "Avoiding Laboratory Test Misinterpretation in Geriatric Rheumatology," *Geriatrics* 44, no. 2 (February 1989): 61–77.

25. Fran Pollner, *Medical World News* 31 (December 1990): 12–13.

26. Lawrence K. Altman, "Electronic Monitoring Doesn't Help in Premature Births, a Study Finds," *New York Times*, March 1, 1990, B10.

27. Benjamin P. Sachs et al., "Sounding Board: Home Monitoring of Uterine Activity: Does It Prevent Prematurity?" *New England Journal of Medicine* 325, no. 19 (November 7, 1991): 1374–78.

28. Lillian Yin, "A Response from the FDA," *New England Journal of Medicine* 325, no. 19 (November 7, 1991): 1377.

29. Julia Bland, "Screeners' Lament," *British Medical Journal* 297 (July 16, 1988): 159–60.

CHAPTER 4. *The Players and the Payers*

1. Richard Davidson, "Source of Funding and Outcome of Clinical Trials," *Journal of General Internal Medicine* 1 (1986): 155–58.

2. Lawrence K. Altman, "Little-Known Doctor Who Found New Use for Common Aspirin," *New York Times*, July 9, 1991, C3.

3. Philippa J. Easterbrook et al., "Publication Bias in Clinical Research," *Lancet* 337, no. 8746 (April 13, 1991): 867–72.

4. Samuel Shapiro, "The Decision to Publish, Ethical Dilemmas," *Journal of Chronic Diseases* 38, no. 4 (1985): 365–72.

5. Lawrence K. Altman, "Hidden Discord Over Right Therapy," *New York Times*, December 24, 1991, C3.

6. Drummond Rennie, "The Cantekin Affair," *Journal of the American Medical Association* 266, no. 23 (December 18, 1991): 3333–37.

7. Jonathan R. Cole, "The Media and Medicine: Believe What You Read at Your Own Risk," *Columbia Magazine*, December 1984, 19–22.

8. David P. Phillips et al., "Importance of the Lay Press in the Transmission of Medical Knowledge to the Scientific Community," *New England Journal of Medicine* 325, no. 16 (October 17, 1991): 1180–83.

9. Deirdre Carmody, "Coverage of Smoking Linked to Tobacco Ads," *New York Times*, January 30, 1992, D22.

10. Randall Rothenberg, "F.D.A. to Scrutinize Drug Makers' Videos," *New York Times*, August 22, 1991, D1.

11. Jim Mitchell, Letter, "And Now, a Word from Our Doctor," *New York Times*, November 17, 1991, 4.

12. Edward D. Freis, "Rationale Against the Drug Treatment of Marginal Diastolic Systemic Hypertension," *American Journal of Cardiology* 66 (August 1, 1990): 368–371.

13. Petr Skrabanek, "Why Is Preventive Medicine Exempted from Ethical Constraints?" *Journal of Medical Ethics* 16 (1990): 187–90.

14. Gill Williams, "Health Promotion—Caring Concern or Slick Salesmanship?" *Journal of Medical Ethics* 10 (1984): 191–95.

15. Michael Kaplan, "Is Your M.D. Being Bribed?" *Self*, March 1991, 168.

16. David A. Kessler, "Drug Promotion and Scientific Exchange: The Role of the Clinical Investigator," *New England Journal of Medicine* 325, no. 3 (July 18, 1991): 201–03.

17. Marjorie A. Bowman, "The Impact of Drug Company Funding on the Content of Continuing Medical Education," *Mobius* 6, no. 1 (January 1986): 66–69.

18. Joel Lexchin, "Advertising Drugs to the Public," *Lancet* (June 17, 1989): 1392–93.

19. James Owen Drife, "Thirty Minutes of Hormone Replacement Therapy," *British Medical Journal* 300 (January 20, 1990).

20. Kumar K. Mehta, Bernard A. Sorofman, and Clayton R. Rowland, *Soc. Sci. Med.* 29, no. 7: 853–57.

21. T. A. French, "Commercial Approach of Pharmaceutical Industry," *British Medical Journal* 287 (November 26, 1983): 1632.

22. Jerry Avorn, Milton Chen, and Robert Hartley, "Scientific versus Commercial Sources of Influence on the Prescribing Behavior of Physicians," *American Journal of Medicine* 73 (July 1982): 4–8.

23. Michael S. Wilkes, Bruce H. Doblin, and Martin F. Shapiro, "Pharmaceutical Advertisements in Leading Medical Journals: Experts' Assessments," *Annals of Internal Medicine* 116, no. 11 (June 1, 1992): 912–919.

24. Judy Ismach, "JAMA's Prescription for Gail McBridge: Two Aspirins and Separation Pay," *Sciencewriters*, April 1984.

25. Elisabeth Rosenthal, "Drug Makers Set Off a Bitter Debate with Ads Aimed Directly at Patients," *New York Times* National, March 3, 1990, 34.

26. Marilyn C. Kincaid, Letter, "Direct-to-Consumer Advertising with Added Inducements," *Journal of the American Medical Association* 267, no. 4 (January 22/29, 1992): 508.

27. Ralph D. Lach, Letter, "The Cholesterol Wars, *Ohio Medicine* (March 1990): 164–65.

28. Jerry Avorn, Daniel E. Everitt, and Merl W. Baker, "The Neglected Medical History and Therapeutic Choices for Abdominal Pain," *Archives of Internal Medicine* 151 (April 1991): 694–98.

29. *West Side Spirit*, September 23, 1985, 4.

30. Richard J. Feinstein, "Medical Scams and Physician Entrepreneurs," *Journal of the Florida Medical Association* 76, no. 5 (May 1989): 436–37.

31. Robert D. Carl III, Letter, "The Doctors' Slice," *New York Times*, May 15, 1991, A26.

32. Robert Pear, with Erik Eckholm, "When Healers Are Entrepre-

neurs: A Debate Over Costs and Ethics," *New York Times*, June 2, 1991, 1.

33. "Rules for Physicians," *Newsday*, September 5, 1991, 16.

34. Robert A. Berenson, "When Opportunity Knocks," *Hastings Center Report*, November/December 1990, 33–35.

35. H. B. Soloway, "Patient-initiated Laboratory Testing: Applauding the Inevitable," *Journal of the American Medical Association* 264 (1990): 1718.

36. Henry B. Soloway, Letter, "Patient-Initiated Laboratory Testing: No Gatekeeper, No Kidding," *Journal of the American Medical Association* 265, no. 4 (January 23/30, 1991): 457–58.

37. Laura Clark, "Are You Seeing Your Fair Share of Patients?" *Medical Economics* 67 (December 10, 1990): 85–93.

38. Mark J. Prashker and Robert F. Meenan, "Subspecialty Training: Is It Financially Worthwhile?" *Annals of Internal Medicine* 115 (1991): 715–19.

39. "Bush Backs Off on Medicare Cuts," *New York Newsday*, August 28, 1991, 17.

40. Letter, "The Health Care Industry: Where Is It Taking Us?" *New England Journal of Medicine* 326, no. 3 (January 16, 1992): 205–07.

41. Walter W. Benjamin, "Sounding Board: Will Centrifugal Forces Destroy the Medical Profession?" *New England Journal of Medicine*, October 26, 1989, 1191–92.

42. Milt Freudenheim, "Debate Widens Over Expanding Use and Growing Costs of Medical Tests, *New York Times*, Saturday, May 30, 1987, p. 49.

43. Brochure from Life Sciences, Inc.

44. Morris Wizenberg, Letter, "Technology Assessment and the Fear of Litigation," *Journal of the American Medical Association* 265, no. 1 (January 2, 1991): 29.

45. A. Russell Localio et al., "Relation Between Malpractice Claims and Adverse Events Due to Negligence," *New England Journal of Medicine* 325, no. 4 (July 25, 1991): 245–51.

46. Stephen B. Thacker and H. David Banta, Letter, "Technology Assessment and the Fear of Litigation," *Journal of the American Medical Association* 265, no. 1 (1991): 29.

47. Arno Vosk, "New Stratagems for Dealing With Medicare's Prospective Payment System and Other Cost-Containment Measures," *Journal of the American Medical Association* 266, no. 1 (July 3, 1991): 121–22.

48. William Murphy, "Hospital Offers Bounty: Rescue Crews Due a Bonus for Patients," *Newsday*, October 29, 1991, 5.

49. Donald W. Simborg, "Sounding Board: DRG Creep: A New Hospital-Acquired Disease," *New England Journal of Medicine* 304 (June 25, 1981): 1602–04.

50. Dorothy Thompson, "Is This the Way We Want to Go?" *British Medical Journal* 302 (March 30, 1991): 795.

51. Lisa Iezzoni et al., "Coding of Acute Myocardial Infarction:

Clinical and Policy Implications," *Annals of Internal Medicine* 109 (November 1, 1988): 745–51.

52. Arthur C. Sturm, Jr., "Signs Show Major Changes Are in Store for Hospitals' Bypass Surgery Business," *Modern Healthcare* (September 23, 1988): 80.

53. C. Brian Spraberry, "Health Care Marketing Minicase: Developing Integrated Referral Channels for Cardiology Services," *Journal of Health Care Marketing* 10, no. 2 (June 1990): 59–61.

54. E. Haavi Morreim, "The New Economics of Medicine: Special Challenges for Psychiatry," *Journal of Medicine and Philosophy* 15 (1990): 97–119.

55. David M. Eddy et al., "The Value of Mammography Screening in Women Under Age 50 Years," *Journal of the American Medical Association* 259, no. 10 (March 11, 1988): 1512–19.

56. Editorial: "Breast Cancer Screening in Women Under 50," *Lancet* 337 (June 29, 1991): 1575–76.

57. Harvey McConnell, "No One Wants to Admit Drug Use Down: Turner," *The Journal* (Addiction Research Foundation of Ontario) (December 1991/January 1992): 3.

58. Barry Werth, "How Short Is Too Short?" *New York Times Magazine*, June 16, 1991, 14–17.

59. Harvey McConnell, "'Sick' Behaviors," *The Journal* (Addiction Research Foundation of Ontario) (January 1, 1989): 16.

60. Erik Eckholm, "Health Benefits Found to Deter Job Switching," *New York Times*, April 28, 1991, 15.

61. Joyce R. Adamson, Letter, "Health Insurers' Rules May Prompt Unnecessary Testing," *Archives of Internal Medicine* 151 (July 1991): 1463.

CHAPTER 5. *Disease-Mongering Tactics*

1. Melvin A. Block, "They Call It Competition," *Archives of Surgery* 124 (July 1989): 771–77.

2. Henry Allen, "America the Bummed," *Newsday*, December 4, 1990.

3. Committee on Safety of Medicine, "Spironolactone," *Current Problems* 21 (January 1988); Gerard S. Conway and Howard S. Jacobs, "Hirsutism," *British Medical Journal* 301 (September 29, 1990): 619–20.

4. "CNS Factsheet: Stress and the Ability to Cope: Powerful Influences on Physical Health," Upjohn News Release, from Manning, Selvage & Lee, Inc., August, 1983.

5. Paul R. Overhulse, Letter, "The Cesarean Section Rates," *Journal of the American Medical Association* 264, no. 8 (August 22/29, 1990): 971.

6. Jean-Charles Sournia, *Ces malades qu'on fabrique*, Paris: (Seuil 1977).

7. *Medical News Tips*, Wang Associates, February 1991.

8. Minerva, "Views," *British Medical Journal*, November 10, 1979, 1231.

9. Barry M. Sherman, Letter, *New York Times Magazine*, July 7, 1991, 4.

10. Kathy Grantham, "Time to Look at Lyme," *North County News*, May 22–May 28, 1991, V4–V7.

11. Alasdair Breckenridge, Editorial: "Treating Mild Hypertension," *British Medical Journal* 291, no. 6488 (July 13, 1985): 89–90.

12. Michael H. Alderman et al., "Antihypertensive Drug Therapy Withdrawal in a General Population," *Archives of Internal Medicine* 146 (July 1986): 1309–11.

13. Fran Pollner, "Panel Waves ERT Closer to Labeling as Heart-Saver," *Medical World News* 31 (July 1990): 46–47.

14. Jonathan R. Cole, "The Media and Medicine: Believe What You Read at Your Own Risk," *Columbia*, December 1984, 19–22.

15. T. G. Pickering, "Treatment of Mild Hypertension and the Reduction of Cardiovascular Mortality: The 'of' or 'by' Dilemma," *Journal of the American Medical Association* 249 (1983): 399–400.

16. Sandra Coney, "New Zealand: Pharmaceutical Advertising," *Lancet* (May 20, 1989): 1128–29.

17. Elaine Blume, Letter, "A Switch in Times Saves a Statistical Bind," *Journal of the American Medical Association* 266, no. 23 (December 18, 1991): 3284.

18. Joseph C. Noreika, "Flu, Indeed! The Dangers of Health-care Advertising," *Journal of the Ohio State Medical Association* (May 1990).

19. Juliet Draper and Martin Roland, "Perimenopausal Women's Views on Taking Hormone Replacement Therapy to Prevent Osteoporosis," *British Medical Journal* 300 (1990): 786–88.

20. Letter, "Perimenopausal Women's Views on Hormone Replacement Therapy," *British Medical Journal* 300 (May 5, 1990): 1196.

21. Press release from E. R. Squibb & Sons.

22. Mike Scott, *A Cognitive-Behavioral Approach to Clients"Problems*, (London: Tavistock/Routledge, 1989).

CHAPTER 6. *Aches and Pains: Becoming a Patient*

1. Marie R. Griffin et al., "Nonsteroidal Anti-inflammatory Drug Use and Increased Risk for Peptic Ulcer Disease in Elderly Persons," *Annals of Internal Medicine* 15 (February 1991): 257–63.

2. S. R. Ahmad, "USA: Crackdown on Misleading Drug Advertising," *Lancet* 338 (November 30, 1991): 1384–85.

3. Nortin M. Hadler, Editorial: "There's the Forest. The Object Lesson of NSAID 'Gastropathy,'" *Journal of Rheumatology* 17, no. 3 (1990): 280–82.

4. Roger A. Renfrew, Letter, "Prevention of NSAID-induced Gastric Ulcer," *Annals of Internal Medicine* 115, no. 11 (December 1, 1991): 912–13.

5. Michael Cherington et al., "Surgery for Thoracic Outlet Syn-

drome May Be Hazardous to Your Health," *Muscle & Nerve* 9 (September 1986): 632.

6. E. C. Hammond, "Some Preliminary Findings on Physical Complaints from a Prospective Study of 1,064,004 Men and Women," *American Journal of Public Health* 54 (1964): 11.

7. K. Dunnell and A. Cartwright, *Medicine Takers, Prescribers and Hoarders* (London: Routledge & Kegan Paul, 1972).

8. Lois M. Vergrugge and Frank J. Ascione, "Exploring the Iceberg: Common Symptoms and How People Care for Them," *Medical Care* 25, no. 6 (June 1987): 539–70.

9. E. M. Brody and M. H. Kleban, "Day-to-Day Mental and Physical Health Symptoms of Older People: A Report on Health Logs," *The Gerontologist* (1983): 23:75.

10. Richard Mayou, Editorial: "Medically Unexplained Physical Symptoms," *British Medical Journal* 303 (September 7, 1991): 534–35.

11. Daniel Goleman, "Patients Refusing to Be Well: A Disease of Many Symptoms," *New York Times* Health, August 21, 1991, C10.

12. Paul Cotton, "Parents' Behavior May Lead Irritable Bowel Syndrome Patients into Physicians' Offices," *Journal of the American Medical Association* 266, no. 3 (July 17, 1991): 317–18.

13. James W. Pennebaker, *The Psychology of Physical Symptoms* (New York: Springer Verlag, 1982).

14. David Mechanic, "Social Psychologic Factors Affecting the Presentation of Bodily Complaints," *New England Journal of Medicine* 286, no. 21 (May 25, 1972): 1132–39.

15. Mark G. Kortepeter, Letter, "MRI: My Resonant Image," *Annals of Internal Medicine* 115, no. 9 (November 1, 1991): 749–50.

16. Sidney R. Block, "Fibrositis and the Concept of Generalized Rheumatism: The Confessions of an Unrepentant Lumper; Nortin M. Hadler, "The Plight of the Patient Whose Illness Is Labeled as Fibrositis or a Related Paralogism," *Occupational Problems in Medical Practice* 5, issue 3.

17. Nortin M. Hadler, "Cumulative Trauma Disorders: An Iatrogenic Concept," *Journal of Occupational Medicine*, 32, no. 1, (January 1990): 38–41.

18. Martin G. Cherniack, "Raynaud's Phenomenon of Occupational Origin," *Archives of Internal Medicine* 150 (March 1990): 519–22.

19. Jerry J. Jasinowski, "Quality Control for Health Care," *New York Times* Forum, March 11, 1990, 13.

20. Nortin M. Hadler, "Regional Musculoskeletal Diseases of the Low Back," *Clinical Orthopaedics and Related Research*, no. 221 (August 1987): 33–41.

21. Marty Goldensohn, "Back Doctors Are a Pain in the Neck!" *Newsday*, January 7, 1992, 68.

22. Albert C. Cuetter and David M. Bartoszek, "The Thoracic Outlet Syndrome: Controversies, Overdiagnosis, Overtreatment, and Recommendations for Management," *Muscle & Nerve*, May 1989, pp. 410–419.

23. Michael Cherington, Letter, "Surgery for Thoracic Outlet Syndrome?" *New England Journal of Medicine* 314 (January 30, 1986): 322.

24. M. Cherington and C. Cherington, "Thoracic Outlet Syndrome: Reimbursement Patterns," *Muscle & Nerve* (September 1991): 897–98.

25. Dean S. Louis, "Cumulative Trauma Disorders," *Journal of Hand Surgery* 12A, no. 5 (September 1987): 823–25.

CHAPTER 7. *Lyme Disease and "Lime" Disease*

1. Joel Lang, "Catching the Bug," *Arthritis Today* (May-June 1988): 43–47.

2. P. Goubau and G. Bigaignon, "Lyme Borreliosis: The New Face of an Old Disease," *Acta Clinica Belgica* 42, no. 1 (1987): 1–4.

3. "Imported Malaria Associated with Malariotherapy of Lyme Disease—New Jersey," *Journal of the American Medical Association* 265, no. 3 (January 16, 1991): 317–18.

4. Ludwig A. Lettau, "Lime Disease—United States," *Annals of Internal Medicine* 114, no. 7 (April 1991): 602.

5. Gregory M. Caputo, Letter, "Lyme Anxiety," *Journal of the American Medical Association* 266, no. 3 (July 17, 1991): 359.

6. Lawrence K. Altman, "Genetic Factor Emerges as Key to Onset of Lyme Arthritis," *New York Times*, July 3, 1990, C1.

7. Kathy Grantham, "Time to Look at Lyme," *North County News*, May 22–May 28, 1991.

8. David Zinman, "Rx for Controversy," *Newsday*, August 6, 1991, 55.

9. Daniel W. Rahn and Stephen E. Malawista, "Lyme Disease: Recommendations for Diagnosis and Treatment," *Annals of Internal Medicine* 114 (1991): 472–81.

10. Brian S. Schwartz et al., "Antibody Testing in Lyme Disease: A Comparison of Results in Four Laboratories," *Journal of the American Medical Association* 262, no. 24 (December 22/29, 1989): 3431–34.

11. Leonard H. Sigal, "Summary of the First 100 Patients Seen at a Lyme Disease Referral Center," *American Journal of Medicine* 88 (June 1990): 577–81.

12. Jane E. Brody, "Personal Health," *New York Times* Health, June 30, 1988, B8.

13. Jane E. Brody, "Personal Health," *New York Times* Health, June 26, 1991, C9.

14. "Plateau Reached at 8,000 Cases in Yearly Reports of Lyme Disease," *New York Times*, June 28, 1991, A16.

15. Daniel S. Berman and Barry D. Wenglin, "Lime Versus Lyme Disease," *Annals of Internal Medicine* 115, no. (July 15, 1991): 158.

16. Alvaro J. Lopez, et al., "Ceftriaxone-induced Cholelithiasis," *Annals of Internal Medicine*, 115, no. 9 (November 1, 1991): 712–14.

CHAPTER 8. *If You're Tired, You Have . . .*

1. Nortin M. Hadler, "Regional Musculoskeletal Diseases of the

Low Back," *Clinical Orthopedics and Related Research*, 221, (August 1987): 33–41.

2. Neenyah Ostrom, *What Really Killed Gilda Radner? Frontline Reports on the Chronic Fatigue Syndrome Epidemic* (New York: That New Magazine, 1991).

3. D. Buchwald, H. Sullivan, and A. L. Komroff, "Frequency of "chronic active Epstein-Barr virus infection" in a general medical practice," *Journal of the American Medical Association* 257 (1987): 2303–2307.

4. Pierre Pichot, *A Century of Psychiatry* (Paris: Editions Roger Dacosta, 1983).

5. G. P. Holmes, *The Chronic Fatigue Syndrome: Definition and Diagnosis* [Proceedings of the Symposium Chronic Fatigue Syndrome, Marseille, France, April 20, 1990] (Paris: Springer-Verlag, 1991).

6. "Chronic Fatigue Syndrome Gains Respect of the Doctors It Thwarts," *New York Times*, December 4, 1990, C1.

7. R. B. Layzer, "Clinical Symptoms in the Chronic Fatigue Syndrome," [Proceedings of the Symposium "Chronic Fatigue Syndrome," Marseille, France, April 20, 1990] (Paris: Springer-Verlag, 1991).

8. Richard D. Huhn, Letter, "Lime Disease," *Annals of Internal Medicine* 115, no. 6 (September 15, 1991): 500.

CHAPTER 9. *Allergy to Life and Everything Else*

1. Don L. Jewett, George Fein, and Martin H. Greenberg, "A Double-Blind Study of Symptom Provocation to Determine Food Sensitivity," *New England Journal of Medicine* 323, no. 7 (August 16, 1990): 429–33.

2. John C. Selner and Herman Staudenmayer, "The Relationship of the Environment and Food to Allergic and Psychiatric Illness," *Psychobiological Aspects of Allergic Disorders*, Stuart H. Young, James M. Rubin, and Harlan R. Daman, Eds. (New York: Praeger 1986).

3. Karen Freifeld and Linda Stasi, "No, It's Not a Tumor, It's a Bread Allergy," *Newsday*, January 23, 1990, [New York] 11.

4. W. E. Dismukes et al., "A Randomized, Double-Blind Trial of Nystatin Therapy for the Candidiasis Hypersensitivity Syndrome," *New England Journal of Medicine* 323 (1990): 1717–23.

5. Gunnar B. Stickler, "I Have an Allergy," *Clinical Pediatrics* (April 1985): 209.

6. T. J. David, "Reactions to Dietary Tartrazine," *Archives of Disease in Childhood* 62 (1987): 119–22.

CHAPTER 10. *Creating Cardiac Cripples I: "Silent" Myocardial Ischemia*

1. Irene Fischl, "The Miracle Peddlers," *New England Journal of Medicine* 321, no. 20 (November 16, 1989): 1417.

2. Thomas B. Graboys, "Conflicts of Interest in the Management

of Silent Ischemia," *Journal of the American Medical Association* 261 (April 14, 1989): 2116–17.

3. Adrian J. B. Brady and John B. Warren, Editorial: "Angioplasty and Restenosis: Endothelium Remains the Sticking Point," *British Medical Journal* 303 (September 28, 1991): 729–30.

4. Sandra Blakeslee, "Defective Warning System Tied to 'Silent' Heart Disease," *New York Times*, May 21, 1985, C1.

5. *Health United States 1990* (Hyattsville, MD: U.S. Department of Health and Human Services, 1991), DHHS Pub. No. (PHS) 91-1232.

6. Graboys, "Conflicts of Interest."

7. Jane E. Brody, "'Silent Heart Disease, a Painless Condition That Poses Great Peril for Millions of Americans," *New York Times* Health, February 21, 1991, B9.

8. S. E. Epstein, A. A. Quyyumi and R. O. Bonow, "Sudden Cardiac Death Without Warning: Possible Mechanisms and Implications for Screening Asymptomatic Populations," *New England Journal of Medicine* 321 (1989): 320–24.

9. Lawrence K. Altman, "Anxiety Linked to Some Chest Pain Cases," *New York Times* Health, August 18, 1988, B12.

10. Francis J. Kane, Jr., Ellison Wittels, and Robert G. Harper, "Chest Pain and Anxiety Disorder," *Journal of Texas Medicine* 86, no. 7 (July 1990): 104–10.

11. Prakash C. Deedwania and Enrique V. Carbajal, "Silent Myocardial Ischemia: A Clinical Perspective," *Archives of Internal Medicine* 151 (December 1991): 2373–82.

12. The following article is reprinted courtesy of *Sports Illustrated* from the May 20, 1985 issue. Copyright © 1985, Time, Inc. ("The Telltale Heart," by Dan Levin.) All rights reserved.

13. Mitchell L. Zoler, "Detecting Asymptomatic CAD: Exercise Tests," *Medical World News* 31 (November 1990): 24–30.

14. Bernard Gutin, "Basic Principles of Training and Fitness," *Active Woman, Contemporary OB-GYN*, May, 1985.

15. Sandra Blakeslee, "Study Links Emotions to Second Heart Attacks," *New York Times*, September 20, 1990.

16. G. Bennett, Letter, "Misleading Exercise Electrocardiograms," *British Medical Journal* 295 (November 7, 1987): 1207.

17. Zoler, "Detecting Asymptomatic CAD."

18. Jay D. Coffman, Editorial: "Intermittent Claudication—Be Conservative," *New England Journal of Medicine* 325, no. 8 (August 22, 1991): 577–78.

19. *Health United States 1990.*

20. Christopher Zarins, "The Vascular War of 1988: The Enemy Is Met," *Journal of the American Medical Association* 261, no. 3 (January 20, 1989): 416–17.

21. Sean R. Tunis et al., "The Use of Angioplasty, Bypass Surgery, and Amputation in the Management of Peripheral Vascular Disease," *New England Journal of Medicine* 325, no. 8 (August 22, 1991): 556–62.

22. Coffman, Editorial.

23. T. J. Ryan et al., "Guidelines for Percutaneous Transluminal Coronary Angioplasty. A Report of the American College of Cardiology/American Heart Association Task Force on Assessment of Diagnostic and Therapeutic Cardiovascular Procedures (Subcommittee on Percutaneous Transluminal Coronary Angioplasty). *Journal of the American College of Cardiology* 12 (1988): 529–45; Robert L. Frye, "President's Page: Role of the Cardiologist in Peripheral Vascular Disease," *Journal of the American College of Cardiology* 18, no. 2 (August 1991): 641–42.

24. D. Eugene Strandness, Jr. et al., "Indiscriminate Use of Laser Angioplasty," *Radiology* 172 (September 1989): 945–46.

25. Ryan et al., "Guidelines."

26. Strandness et al., "Indiscriminate Use."

27. Victor Gurewich, Letter, "The Vascular War," *Journal of the American Medical Association* 261, no. 24 (June 23/30, 1989): 3550.

28. Zarins, "The Vascular War of 1988."

CHAPTER 11. *Creating Cardiac Cripples II: Murmurs, Mitral Valve Prolapse and Arrhythmias*

1. Susan Walton, Hers column, *New York Times*, June 25, 1987, C2.

2. A. C. Doyle, "The Sign of Four," in *The Complete Sherlock Holmes* (New York: Doubleday, 1930), 100.

3. Donald Janson, "Heart Attack Kills Boy During Soccer Practice," *New York Times*, September 26, 1985.

4. Dan G. McNamara, Letter, "Avoiding Anxiety About 'Innocent' Heart Murmur," *American Journal of Diseases of Children* 142 (June 1988): 587.

5. Basanti Mukerji, Martin A. Alpert, and Vaskar Mukerji, "Cardiovascular Changes in Athletes," *American Family Physician* (September 1989): 169–75.

6. Gunnar B. Stickler, "The Fear of Recording a Negative Physical Examination," *European Journal of Pediatrics* 137 (1981): 3–4.

7. Frank Gross, Letter: "The Emperor's Clothes Syndrome," *New England Journal of Medicine* 285, no. 15 (October 7, 1971): 863.

8. Abraham B. Bergman, "Controlling Iatrogenic Diseases," *Israel Journal Med. S.* 15, no. 3 (March 1979): 199.

9. G. G. Cayler, D. B. Lynn, and E. M. Stein, "Effect of Cardiac Nondisease on Intellectual and Perceptual Motor Development," *British Heart Journal* 35 (1973): 543–47.

10. Noble O. Fowler, *Diagnosis of Heart Disease* (New York: Springer Verlag, 1991): 46.

11. Joseph D. Wassersug, "Never Shrug Off the Reason the Patient Came to See You," *Medical Economics* (December 10, 1990): 97–98.

12. Jane E. Brody, "Personal Health," *New York Times*, March 28, 1991, B11.

13. Richard B. Devereux, Editorial: "Diagnosis and Prognosis of

Mitral-Valve Prolapse," *New England Journal of Medicine* 320, no. 16 (April 20, 1989): 1077–79.

14. S. W. MacMahon et al., "Risk of Infective Endocarditis in Mitral Valve Prolapse With and Without Precoridal Systolic Murmurs, *American Journal of Cardiology* 59 (January 1, 1987): 105–08.

15. Aubrey Leatham and Wallace Brigden, "Mild Mitral Regurgitation and the Mitral Prolapse Fiasco," *American Heart Journal*, 99, no. 5 (May 1980): 659–64.

16. Donald Kaye and Elias Abrutyn, Editorial: "Prevention of Bacterial Endocarditis: 1991," *Annals of Internal Medicine* 114, no. 9 (May 1, 1991): 803–04.

17. Richard B. Devereux, "Diagnosis and Prognosis of Mitral-Valve Prolapse," *New England Journal of Medicine* 320, no. 16 (April 20, 1989): 1077–79.

18. *American Heart Journal* 113 (February 1987): 341.

19. Joshua Wynne, Editorial: "Mitral-Valve Prolapse," *New England Journal of Medicine* 314, no. 9 (February 27, 1986): 577–78.

20. Richard B. Devereux et al., "Relation Between Clinical Features of the Mitral Prolapse Syndrome and Echocardiographically Documented Mitral Valve Prolapse," *Journal of the American College of Cardiology* 8 (1986): 763–72.

21. Timothy E. Quill, Mack Lipkin, Jr., and Philip Greenland, "The Medicalization of Normal Variants: The Case of Mitral Valve Prolapse," *Journal of General Internal Medicine* 3 (May-June 1988): 267–76.

22. James J. Lynch et al., "Human Contact and Cardiac Arrhythmias in a Coronary Care Unit," *Psychosomatic Medicine* 39, no. 3 (May-June 1977): 188–92.

23. L. K. Hine, T. P. Gross, and D. L. Kennedy. "Outpatient Antiarrhythmic Drug Use from 1970 Through 1986." *Archives of Internal Medicine* 149 (1989): 1524–27.

24. "The Cardiac Arrhythmia Suppression Trial (CAST). Preliminary Report: Effect of Encainide and Flecainide on Mortality in a Randomized Trial of Arrhythmia Suppression After Myocardial Infarction," *New England Journal of Medicine* 321 (1989): 406–12.

25. Joel Morganroth, J. Thomas Bigger, Jr., and Jeffrey L. Anderson, "Treatment of Ventricular Arrhythmias by United States Cardiologists: A Survey Before the Cardiac Arrhythmia Suppression Trial Results Were Available," *American Journal of Cardiology* 65 (January 1, 1990): 40–48.

26. James W. Mold and Howard F. Stein, "Sounding Board: The Cascade Effect in the Clinical Care of Patients," *New England Journal of Medicine* 314, no. 8 (February 20, 1986): 512–14.

27. Stickler, "The Fear of Recording."

CHAPTER 12. *The "Diseasing" of Risk Factors: High Cholesterol and Blood Pressure*

1. Thomas Moore, *Heart Failure* (New York: Random House, 1989).

2. Russell Baker, "Observer: The Cholesterol Thing," *New York Times*, November 29, 1989, A31.

3. Alasdair Breckenridge, "Treating Mild Hypertension," *British Medical Journal* 291, no. 6488 (July 13, 1985): 89–90.

4. S. G. Thompson and S. J. Popcock, "The Variability of Serum Cholesterol Measurements: Implications for Screening and Monitoring," *Journal of Clinical Epidemiology* 43, no. 8 (1990): 783–89.

5. "High Cholesterol Threatening Many," *New York Times*, November 28, 1986.

6. James H. Warram et al., "Excess Mortality Associated with Diuretic Therapy in Diabetes Mellitus," *Archives of Internal Medicine* 151 (July 1991): 1350–56.

7. Einar T. Skarfors, K. Ingemar Selinus, and Hans O. Lithell, "Risk Factors for Developing Non-Insulin Dependent Diabetes: A 10-Year Follow-Up of Men in Uppsala," *British Medical Journal* 303 (September 28, 1991): 755–60.

8. Michael H. Criqui, "Cholesterol, Primary and Secondary Prevention, and All-Cause Mortality," *Annals of Internal Medicine* 115, no. 12 (December 15, 1991): 973–76.

9. Tony Delamothe, "Consensus on Cholesterol," *British Medical Journal*, 302 (April 6, 1991): 806.

10. T. E. Strandberg et al., "Long Term Mortality After 5 Year Multifactorial Primary Prevention of Cardiovascular Diseases in Middle Aged Men," *Journal of the American Medical Association* 226 (1991): 1225–29.

11. Philip M. Boffey, "Cholesterol: Debate Flares Over Wisdom in Widespread Reductions," *New York Times* (Science Times), July 14, 1987, C1.

12. Allan S. Brett, "Treating Hypercholesterolemia: How Should Practicing Physicians Interpret the Published Data for Patients?" *New England Journal of Medicine* 321, no. 10 (September 7, 1989) 676–80.

13. Lipid Research Clinics Program, "The Lipid Research Clinics Coronary Primary Prevention Trial Results," *Journal of the American Medical Association* 251, no. 3 (January 20, 1984): 351–74.

14. Jonathan R. Cole, "The Media and Medicine: Believe What You Read at Your Own Risk," *Columbia Magazine*, December 1984, 19–22.

15. Stephen B. Hulley and Andrew L. Avins, "Asymptomatic Hypertriglyceridaemia," *British Medical Journal* 304 (February 15, 1992): 393–96.

16. W. C. Taylor et al., "Cholesterol Reduction and Life Expectancy: A Model Incorporating Multiple Risk Factors. *Annals of Internal Medicine* 106 (April 1987): 605–14.

17. P. C. Elwood, Letter, "Lowering Cholesterol Concentrations and Mortality," *British Medical Journal* 301 (October 20, 1990): 930.

18. Warren S. Browner, Janice Westenhouse, and Jeffrey A. Tice, "What If Americans Ate Less Fat? A Quantitative Estimate of the Effect

on Mortality," *Journal of the American Medical Association* 265, no. 24 (June 26, 1991): 3285–91.

19. Hal B. Richerson, Letter, *New England Journal of Medicine* 324, no. 1 (January 3, 1991): 61.

20. "Conversation with Sir Richard Doll," *British Journal of Addiction* 86 (1991): 365–77.

21. Gina Kolata, "Major Study Aims to Learn Who Should Lower Cholesterol," *New York Times*, September 26, 1989, C1.

22. Warren E. Leary, "Federal Official Faults Public Cholesterol Tests," *New York Times*, November 28, 1989, C8.

23. B. J. Milne, A. G. Logan, and P. T. Flanagan, "Alterations in health perception and lifestyle in created hypertensives," *Journal of Chronic Diseases* 37 (1984): 417–423.

24. R. Brian Haynes et al., "Increased Absenteeism from Work After Detection and Labeling of Hypertensive Patients," *New England Journal of Medicine* 299, no. 14 (October 5, 1978): 741–44.

25. Joan R. Bloom and Susan Monterossa, "Hypertension Labeling and Sense of Well-Being," *American Journal of Public Health* 71, no. 11 (November 1981): 1228–32.

26. Allan S. Brett, "Psychologic Effects of the Diagnosis and Treatment of Hypercholesterolemia: Lessons from Case Studies," *American Journal of Medicine* 91 (December 1991): 642–47.

27. Lynn Payer, *Medicine & Culture* (New York: Henry Holt, 1988).

28. "More on Hypertensive Labelling," *Lancet* (May 18, 1985): 1138–39.

29. Norman M. Kaplan, *Clinical Hypertension* (5th ed.) (Baltimore: Williams and Wilkins, 1990).

30. Robert E. Olson, "Risk Factors for Coronary Heart Disease," *Stony Brook Health Sciences Center Health Letter* 1, no. 4 (September 1989): 1.

31. Richerson, Letter.

32. "High Cholesterol? Maybe. Maybe Not," *Harvard Medical School Health Letter* 12, no. 11 (September 1987): 2.

33. "Body Position Is Found to Affect the Accuracy of Heart Disease Tests," *New York Times*, June 24, 1986, C3.

34. Laurie Garrett, "Report Hits Cholesterol Testing," *Newsday*, November 28, 1989, 17.

35. Brett, "Psychologic Effects."

36. Beth Schucker et al., "Change in Cholesterol Awareness and Action," *Archives of Internal Medicine* 151 (April 1991): 666.

37. Randolph L. Gordon, Michael J. Klag and Paul K. Whelton, "Community Cholesterol Screening: Impact of Labeling on Participant Behavior," *Archives of Internal Medicine* 150 (September 1990): 1957–1960.

38. Thomas B. Newman, Warren S. Browner, and Stephen B. Hulley, "Childhood Cholesterol Screening: Contraindicated," *Journal of the American Medical Association* 267, no. 1 (January 1, 1992): 100–01.

39. Ronald M. Lauer and William B. Clarke, "Use of Cholesterol

Measurements in Childhood for the Prediction of Adult Hypercholesterolemia: The Muscatine Study," *Journal of the American Medical Association* 264 (1990): 3034–38.

40. James E. Dalen, "Detection and Treatment of Elevated Blood Cholesterol: What Have We Learned?" *Archives of Internal Medicine* 151 (January 1991): 25–28.

41. Newman et al., "Childhood Cholesterol."

42. Ralph D. Lach, Letter, "The Cholesterol Wars," *Ohio Medicine* 86 (March 1990): 164–65.

43. Lach Letter.

44. Adam L. Linton and C. David Naylor, "Organized Medicine and the Assessment of Technology: Lessons from Ontario," *New England Journal of Medicine* 323, no. 21 (November 22, 1990): 1463–67.

CHAPTER 13. *The Medicalization of Menopause: Choose Your Disease*

1. "Women Face 1-in-9 Chance of Breast Cancer, Group Says," *New York Times* National, January 25, 1991, A18.

2. Letter, Wang Associate Health Communications, December 26, 1990.

3. Michael Unger, "Antibiotic Heads Prescription List," *Newsday*, February 5, 1991, 33.

4. Julia Kagan and Jo David, "The Facts of Life: What Every Woman Over 35 Needs to Know About Her Body," *McCalls*, June 1991, 60–140.

5. "Systemic Treatment of Early Breast Cancer By Hormonal, Cytotoxic, or Immune Therapy," *Lancet* 339, no. 8784 (January 4, 1992): 1–15.

6. Jane E. Brody, "Personal Health," *New York Times*, February 12, 1992; Lawrence K. Altman, "Study on Breast Cancer Finds Therapy Is Effective for Years," *New York Times*, January 3, 1992, 1.

7. Bernard Shaw, *The Doctor's Dilemma* (Harmondsworth, England: Penguin, 1977).

8. Joseph Palca, "NIH Unveils Plan for Women's Health Project," *Science* 254 (November 8, 1991): 792.

9. Ellen Goodman, "Wanted: A Definitive Answer on Estrogen," *New York Newsday*, September 17, 1991, 82. Copyright 1991, The Boston Globe Newspaper Co./Washington Post Writer's Group. Reprinted with permission.

10. Jan P. Vandenbroucke, "Postmenopausal Oestrogen and Cardioprotection," *Lancet* 337 (April 6, 1991): 833–34.

11. Thomas E. Moon, "Estrogens and Disease Prevention," *Archives of Internal Medicine* 151 (January 1991): 17–18.

12. Lee Goldman and Anna N. A. Tosteson, "Uncertainty About Postmenopausal Estrogen," *New England Journal of Medicine* 325, no. 11 (September 12, 1991): 800–02.

13. Gina Kolata, "Estrogen After Menopause Cuts Heart Attack Risk, Study Finds," *New York Times*, September 12, 1991, 1.

14. Fran Pollner, "Panel Waves ERT Closer to Labeling as Heart-Saver," *Medical World News* (July 1990): 46–47.

15. John E. Sutherland, Victoria W. Persky, and Jacob A. Brody, "Proportionate Mortality Trends: 1950 Through 1986," *Journal of the American Medical Association* 264, no. 24 (December 26, 1990): 3178–84.

16. *Health United States 1990* (Hyattsville, MD: U.S. Department of Health and Human Services, Public Health Service, Centers for Disease Control, National Center for Health Statistics, 1991), DHHS Pub. No. (PHS) 91-1232, 84.

17. L.Tobias Kircher, "Autopsy and Mortality Statistics: Making a Difference," Pulse, *Journal of the American Medical Association*, March 4, 1992, 267, no. 9, 1264–1268.

18. Constance Percy and Alice Dolman, "Comparison of the Coding of Death Certificates Related to Cancer in Seven Countries," *Public Health Reports* 93, no. 4 (July-August 1978): 335–50.

19. L. Bergkuist et al., "The Risk of Breast Cancer After Estrogen and Estrogen-Progestin Replacement," *New England Journal of Medicine* 321 (1989): 293.

20. K. K. Steinberg, S. B. Thacker, S. J. Smith et al., "A Meta-Analysis of the Effect of Estrogen Replacement Therapy on the Risk of Breast Cancer," *Journal of the American Medical Association* 265 (1991): 1985–90.

21. Gina Kolata, "Cancer Experts See a Need for Caution on Use of Birth Pill," *New York Times*, January 7, 1989, 1.

22. "Role of Hormones in Breast-Cancer Risk," *Contemporary OB/GYN* (April 1991): 80–95.

23. "Estrogen Replacement Therapy Safe, Says Hopkins Doctor," The Johns Hopkins Medical Institutions Medical News Tips, March 5, 1991, 2.

24. Michael Davie, Letter, *British Medical Journal* 301, (November 3, 1990): 1017.

CHAPTER 14. *"Precancerous" Breasts and the Overselling of Mammography*

1. Susan M. Love, Rebecca Sue Gelman, and William Silen, "Sounding Board: Fibrocystic 'Disease' of the Breast—A Nondisease?" *New England Journal of Medicine* 307, no. 16 (October 14, 1982): 1010–14.

2. Jeremy Weir Alderson, "An Indecent Proposal," *Mother Jones* (May 1965): 52–56.

3. Susan Love, M.D. with Karen Lindsey, *Dr. Susan Love's Breast Book* (Reading, Mass.: Merloyd Lawrence 1990).

4. Elaine Blume and David Artz, "Too Many Breast Biopsies? Watching vs. Cutting," *Journal of the National Cancer Institute* 83, no. 17 (September 4, 1991): 1207.

5. Robert McLelland, "Supply and Quality of Screening Mammography: A Radiologist's View," *Annals of Internal Medicine* 113, no. 7 (October 1, 1990): 490.

6. Martin L. Brown, Larry G. Kessler, and Fred Rueter, "Is the Supply of Mammography Machines Outstripping Need and Demand," *Annals of Internal Medicine* 113, no. 7 (October 1, 1990): 547–52.

7. Russell P. Harris et al., "Mammography and Age: Are We Targeting the Wrong Women?" *Cancer* 67 (April 1, 1991): 2010–14.

8. "Darts and Laurels," *Columbia Journalism Review* (September-October 1991): 21.

9. Paul C. Stomper et al., "New England Mammography Survey: Public Misconceptions of Breast Cancer Incidence," *Breast Disease* 3 (1990): 7.

10. Sandra Blakeslee, "Faulty Math Heightens Fears of Breast Cancer," *New York Times Week in Review* March 15, 1992, 1.

11. John E. Woods and Phillip G. Arnold, "Terror of Cancer Brings Them to Us," *Wall Street Journal*, February 20, 1992.

12. Vincent R. Pennisi, "We're Losing the War on Breast Cancer," *Wall Street Journal*, January 31, 1992, A15.

13. Susan M. Williams, "Mammography in Women Under Age 30. Is There Clinical Benefit?" *Radiology* 161 (1986): 49–51.

14. Stanley Edeiken, "Mammography and Palpable Cancer of the Breast," *Cancer* 61 (January 15, 1988): 263–65.

15. Ferris M. Hall, Letter, "Mammography in Women Under Age 30: Is There Clinical Benefit?" *Radiology* 162 (February 1987): 582.

16. David M. Eddy et al., "The Value of Mammography Screening in Women Under Age 50 Years," *Journal of the American Medical Association* 259, no. 10 (March 11, 1988): 1512–19.

17. Editorial "Breast Cancer Screening in Women Under 50," *Lancet* 337 (June 29, 1991): 1575–76.

18. Press release, American College of Radiology, March 16, 1990.

19. Susan Love, "Breast Cancer: Early Decisions," *Harvard Medical School Health Letter* (March 1988).

20. Maja Nielsen, Jorn Jensen, and John Andersen, "Precancerous and Cancerous Breast Lesions During Lifetime and at Autopsy: A Study of 83 Women," *Cancer* 54 (1984): 612–15.

21. James J. McCabe, Michele L. Hartigan and Elise E. Singer, "Medicolegal Aspects in Breast Cancer Treatment," *Breast Cancer Treatment*, Barbara Fowble et al., eds. (St. Louis: Mosby Year Book, 1991).

22. Caroline A. Jones, Letter, "More Than Mammography, Self-Examination Detects Cancers," *New York Times*, June 18, 1991, A18.

23. G. J. Lesnick, "Detection of Breast Cancer in Young Women," *Journal of the American Medical Association* 237 (1977): 967–69.

24. Caryn Lerman et al., "Psychological and Behavioral Implications of Abnormal Mammograms," *Annals of Internal Medicine* 114 (1991): 657–61.

25. Blume and Artz, "Too Many Breast Biopsies?"

26. Ruth Warren, Letter, "Team Learning and Breast Cancer Screening," *Lancet* 338 (August 24, 1991): 514.

27. Ann Landers, *New York Newsday*, February 18, 1991, 46.

28. "The Breast Cancer Challenge of 1991," *Journal of the National Cancer Institute* 83, no. 13 (July 3, 1991): 914–15.

29. Polly A. Newcomb et al., "Breast Self-Examination in Relation to the Occurrence of Advanced Breast Cancer," *Journal of the National Cancer Institute* 83, no. 4 (February 20, 1991): 260–65.

CHAPTER 15: *Cosmetic Considerations*

1. Robert M. Goldwyn, "Plastic Surgeons on the Make," *Plastic and Reconstructive Surgery* (83 February 1989): 251–52.

2. Joan E. Rigdon, "Informed Consent? Plastic Surgeons Had Warnings on Safety of Silicone Implants," *Wall Street Journal*, March 12, 1992, 1.

3. Felicity Barringer, "Plastic Surgery: A Profession in Need of a Facelift?" *New York Times*, February 23, 1992, E5.

4. Peter S. Vig, "Orthodontic Controversies: Their Origins, Consequences, and Resolution," *Current Controversies in Orthodontics*, Birle Melsen, ed., (Chicago: Quintessence, 1991).

5. R. Burgersdijk et al., "Community-Dentistry and Oral Epidemiology 19, no. 2 (April 1991): 61–63.

6. Jane Berentson, "Doctors Stress Size Not Risks to a 'Patient,' " *Wall Street Journal*, March 12, 1992, A4.

7. Lois W. Banner, *American Beauty* (New York: Knopf, 1983).

8. Ronald P. Strauss, "Ethical and Social Concerns in Facial Surgical Decision Making," *Plastic and Reconstructive Surgery* 72, no. 5 (November 1983): 727–30.

9. Tamar Lewin, "As Silicone Issue Grows, Women Take Agony and Anger to Court," *New York Times*, January 19, 1992, 1.

10. Sidney M. Wolfe, "Letter," *Wall Street Journal*, January 13, 1992, A15.

11. Joan E. Rigdon, "Informed Consent? Plastic Surgeons Had Warnings on Safety of Silicone Implants," *Wall Street Journal*, March 12, 1992, 1.

12. "After U.S. Warning, Dow Curbs Assurances About Breast Implants," *New York Times*, January 1, 1992, 8.

13. Vincent Canby, "'Barton Fink' Wins the Top Prize and 2 Others at Cannes Festival," *New York Times*, May 21, 1991, C13.

14. C. R. Buchanan, M. A. Preece, and R. D. G. Milner, "Mortality, Neoplasia and Creutzfeldt-Jakob Disease in Patients Treated with Human Pituitary Growth Hormone in the United Kingdom," *British Medical Journal* 302 (April 6, 1991): 824.

15. T. Billette deVillemeur et al., "Creutzfeldt-Jakob Disease in Children Treated with Growth Hormone," *Lancet* 337 (April 6, 1991) 865.

16. J. M. Walker et al., "Treatment of Short Normal Children With Growth Hormone—A Cautionary Tale?" *Lancet* 336 (December 1, 1990) 1331–34.

17. Barry Werth, "How Short Is Too Short?" *New York Times Magazine*, June 16, 1991, 14.

18. Gunnar B. Stickler, "'Failure to Thrive' or the Failure to Define," *Pediatrics* 74 (1984): 559.

19. Gunnar B. Stickler, "Gastrostomy Dependence in Two Constitutionally Short Children," *American Journal of Diseases of Children* 142 (September 1988): 937–39.

20. Marilyn Chase, "Scientists Work to Slow Human Aging," *Wall Street Journal*, March 12, 1992, B1.

21. Don Vaughan, "Hung Up On Size?" *Omni*.

CHAPTER 16. *Psychiatric "Disorders": From Hyperactive Kids to Anxiety and Insomnia*

1. H. P. Rome, "Psychiatry and Foreign Affairs," *American Journal of Psychiatry* 125 (December 1968): 725–30.

2. Roberta C. Redford, Letter, "Bettelheim Became the Very Evil He Loathed," *New York Times*, November 20, 1990, A20.

3. Peter Kerr, "Chain of Mental Hospitals Faces Inquiry in 4 States," *New York Times*, October 22, 1991, 1.

4. Bob Liff, "Alter Seeks Limits on City Psychiatrists," *Newsday*, November 19, 1991, 108.

5. Helen Hershfield Avnet, *Psychiatric Insurance* (New York: Group Health Insurance, 1962): 209–210.

6. Alan A. Lipton and Franklin S. Simon, "Psychiatric Diagnosis in a State Hospital: Manhattan State Revisited," *Hospital and Community Psychiatry* 36, no. 4 (April 1985): 368–73.

7. Daniel Goleman, "State Hospital Accused of Wrong Diagnoses, Fueling Debate Over Nation's Mental Care," *New York Times*, April 23, 1985, C1.

8. E. Haavi Morreim, "The New Economics of Medicine: Special Challenges for Psychiatry," *Journal of Medicine and Philosophy* 15 (1990): 97–119.

9. Jamie Talan, "Psychiatry Pioneer Menninger Dies," *Newsday*, July 19, 1990, 37.

10. Robert Shepherd, "Psychiatry's Shrinking Roots: The Untold Story," *Medical Post*, March 20, 1984, 13.

11. Morreim, "The New Economics of Medicine."

12. L. A. Weithorn, "Mental Hospitalization of Troublesome Youth: An Analysis of Skyrocketing Admission Rates," *Stanford Law Review* 40 (1988): 773–838.

13. "Controversy Still Surrounds ADD," *Lahey Clinic Health Letter*, February, 1992, 5.

14. "What Was Said," *Medical Post*, September 16, 1986, 2.

15. Gabrielle Weiss, "Hyperactivity in Childhood," *New England Journal of Medicine* 323, no. 20 (November 15, 1990): 1413–45.

16. Martha Weinman Lear, "Redefining Anxiety," *The New York Times Magazine*, July 31, 1988, 30.

17. David Mechanic, "Social Psychologic Factors Affecting the Presentation of Bodily Complaints," *New England Journal of Medicine* 286, no. 21 (May 25, 1972): 1132–39.

18. Ian Robertson, "Medicine and the Media: A Near Myth," *British Medical Journal* 302 (February 2, 1991): 297.

19. Ann Landers, *New York Newsday*, April 29, 1991, 44.

20. William Styron, "Pills as Accessories to Depression," *New York Newsday*, July 31, 1991, 79.

21. "Sleeping Just Got Easier," *Medical News Tips* 2, no. 1 (February 1991) Wang Associates.

22. "Rise and Shine," *Medical News Tips*, the Johns Hopkins Medical Institutions.

23. E. O. Bixler et al., "Next-Day Memory Impairment with Triazolam Use," *Lancet* 337 (1991): 827–31.

24. David J. Greenblatt, Richard I. Shader, and Jerold S. Harmatz, Letter, *New England Journal of Medicine* 325, no. 24 (December 12, 1991): 1744.

25. Mark S. Silverman, Letter, "Triazolam in the Elderly," *New England Journal of Medicine* 325, no. 24 (December 12, 1991): 1742.

CHAPTER 17. *Diagnosing Our Genes*

1. Gina Kolata, "Discovery of Worsening Family Ills Spurs Rush to Tap Potential Bonanza," *New York Times*, February 25, 1992, C3.

2. Leslie Roberts, "To Test or Not to Test," *Science* 247 (January 5, 1990): 17–19.

3. Kathryn H. Spitzer and Lytt I. Gardner, Letter, "Genetic Counseling," *Journal of the American Medical Association* 253, no. 2 (January 11, 1985): 202–03.

4. Mitchel L. Zoler, "Genetic Tests," *Medical World News*, January 1991, 32–37.

CHAPTER 18. *Putting Disease In Its Place: A Prescription for Change*

1. William Murphy, "Hospital Offers Bounty: Rescue Crews Due a Bonus for Patients"; Gale Scott, "8-Hour Wait for Treating Patients," *Newsday*, October 29, 1991, 5.

2. John Markoff, "Europe Takes the Lead in Privacy Protection," *New York Times*, April 14, 1991, 9.

3. David C. Hsia, "Qui Tam: Suing Physicians Who Make False Claims," *Annals of Internal Medicine* 114, no. 12 (June 15, 1991): 1050–53.

4. Mitchel L. Zoler, "Genetic Tests," *Medical World News* 32 (January 1991): 32–37.

Index